PHILIP ELLEY

PULL YOURSELF TOGETHER MAN

EMOTIONAL HEALTH ADVICE FOR MEN, AND THOSE THAT KNOW THEM

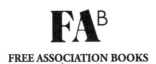

FREE ASSOCIATION BOOKS

First published in 2023 by
Free Association Books

Copyright © 2023 Philip Eley

The author's rights are fully asserted. The right of
Philip Eley to be identified as the author of this work
has been asserted by him in accordance with the
Copyright, Designs and Patents Act 1988

A CIP Catalogue of this book is available from
the British Library

ISBN: 978-19113837-9-6

Cover design and typeset by
www.chandlerbookdesign.com

Printed in Great Britain by
TJ Books Limited, Padstow, Cornwall

CONTENTS

DEDICATION

For my dad, Richard Eley, who showed
me how to be a good man.

Introduction

I'm a man who struggles with my emotional health. Every day I use simple tips and techniques to manage my wellbeing. I've been doing this so long that I've got to the point where I don't even have to think about these things anymore; they have just become effective rhythms and healthy habits in my life.

If I didn't do this, I'd be a complete mess. I'm a bit of a mess now, but then so are all my favourite people. I don't really want to hang out with perfect people. Partly because I don't think perfect people exist, but, even if they did, I don't think they'd be the easiest friends. If you think this book, or any book, will give you a perfect life, think again. There are no magic wands, no genie's lamps, no fairy tale endings. However, I am remarkably content and astonishingly happy. On a scale of one to ten, with one being the lowest I've felt in my life and ten being the maximum state of happiness I've ever reached, I've been above seven for a long time, and I'm happy with that. That's not my natural state. I have struggled with my mental health my whole life, particularly with anxiety, and I was on anti-depressants in my twenties.

But, because I regularly manage my emotional health, I am not held back by any of these things. That's a key for me. I aim to get my wellbeing to a place where it generally pushes me forward, rather than holds me back.

I think that effective rhythms and healthy habits far outweigh circumstances when it comes to affecting our wellbeing. I have travelled a lot, and, if there is one thing I've learned through travel, it's that people in the most difficult circumstances are often the happiest. I don't think circumstances affect our happiness as much as we often think they do.

Pull Yourself Together, Man is written as a simple, usable guide on how to find some effective rhythms and healthy habits in your life. It offers ideas and thoughts to help people better manage their own emotional health. It contains stories, lists and ideas, as well as top tips and anecdotes. I have talked to most of the males I know about their own ways of managing their wellbeing, and I've heard a lot of honesty and a lot of heartbreak. Alongside this, I've also seen a lot of humour and resilience. All these ideas and stories are woven throughout the book. There's also passion there. When men talk about the things and people that they love, they talk with a beautiful passion and intensity. I love to hear about people's passions and how those things affect people's wellbeing, so I have collected some of these stories as well. I've also sat with groups of males and talked in depth about their wellbeing and emotional health. In this way, this book is a collective effort. It is a form of camaraderie, a way of saying that you're not alone; a way of saying that we understand that what you are going through is difficult, and we hope things will get better; a way of sharing some of the thoughts and ideas which have worked for us in an on-going project of finding some wellbeing.

I'm the wellbeing lead of a charity. This job involves some one-to-one listening, some small group work and some emotional health training. My job involves making the complicated simple. The brain is so complicated that we're only just finding out certain things. Wellbeing can be incredibly complicated, but it can be made simple too. Focusing on your own wellbeing is a start. Over years we build up unhealthy habits, and the sooner you start to recognise these unhealthy habits, the more time you have to change them.

I help both men and women with the management and recovery of their emotional health. I've been doing this for many years and in that time I have encountered and developed many ideas, techniques and resources which have helped hundreds of people. Every human is an individual and everyone is different, but I have seen patterns over that time in the ways that some men approach issues around mental health, as opposed to how some women approach the same issues. There is often a different language used and a different approach to accepting help. There might be more reluctance to reach out for help in the first place, and more work to be done in lowering defences and becoming vulnerable. This book is written particularly for those people, only some of whom are men, who find it hard to be vulnerable, and don't know how to ask for help. But it's also written for anyone at all who struggles at times with their emotional health, and that's most of us.

The Hard Facts

Men are three times more likely to intentionally kill themselves than women are.

The statistics are shocking. But, in many ways, it's the personal stories which hit home harder. Most men I know can tell you a story of someone close to them who is struggling. Or worse.

Men are struggling. Name three things which men commonly struggle with.
1.
2.
3.

Why do you think that men are three times more likely to kill themselves than women?

Everyone's emotional health is damaged. That's everyone! No one has perfect emotional health. Our emotional health is damaged by our childhoods, our struggles, our successes, our relationships, our failed relationships, our unfulfilled hopes and dreams, our genes, our habits and much more besides. Our emotional health is tied in with our identity. Sometimes it's hard to know where we end and our struggles begin. And some struggle is necessary. Wellbeing isn't about being perfect and it's not about perpetual happiness. There will always be ups and downs, but all of us could probably do with a few less downs and a few more ups. There are no quick fixes, but there are choices, and patterns and new ways of approaching life which WILL bring some recovery. In the end, finding wellbeing isn't about changing a person, but it is about smoothing some of the more difficult edges. It is about building effective rhythms and healthy habits.

I am surrounded by men who are struggling to cope. Men are struggling in all kinds of circumstances and for all kinds of reasons. Men are struggling with difficult lives and difficult feelings. And sometimes they get told to pull themselves together. This phrase suggests that it is simple to ignore difficult feelings or to distract yourself from them. And in the short term, this is sometimes possible. But this is never a good long-term strategy. People have been throwing this phrase at men in a way that suggests it's simple for too long, and it is not helping. I'm re-claiming this phrase to mean something more fundamental and on-going. Something difficult, but possible.

Have you ever been told to pull yourself together, or man up? How did that feel?

There isn't a person alive who doesn't need emotional health. My job involves helping people with the management and recovery of their emotional health. In this way, there is a sense in which we can pull ourselves together. If we approach the healing process as a long-term project involving emotional health, maintenance and renewal, with the support of other people, then there are things which will generally help us to pull ourselves together. There are practical ways to manage emotional health. Our bodies and brains naturally seek health, and, given the right circumstances, they will find some recovery. There are practical ways of managing emotional health which often bring some relief.

Controversial?

Mental health in general is controversial. It used to carry a stigma, but, thankfully, this is becoming reduced. Instead, the growing controversy focuses around medication. The big question around mental health focuses on whether we diagnose and medicate too easily, particularly with children. As you'd expect, there are vocal groups in both camps. I'm a grey area thinker and I can see both sides. There are no principles or practices in this book which contradict, or support, either side. Everything that I talk about could be used by someone who firmly believed in diagnosis and medication, but just as easily used by someone who didn't.

Who is this book for?

This book is for people who sometimes struggle with difficult emotions. In my experience, that's most of us. Most of us have built up unhealthy thinking habits which hold us back from being the best we can be. This book encourages you to build a healthier emotional approach to life. I talk about this goal as a project. It's not quick, and it's not easy, but it is achievable. All the best projects need a guide, and this book is that guide. A lot of big projects also need additional support and I'd encourage you to find additional support when needed.

A guide for men?

Although this is a guide for men and those who know them, the advice isn't exclusive. When I help people manage their emotional health, I don't have one set of ideas for men and one for women. I've just seen a lot of men struggle and this has prompted me to write a book with these people in mind. I have set out to write a book which will resonate with men I have met, but I have no intention of excluding anyone from the conversation; if these ideas resonate with others too, then that is fantastic.

When I have asked men for their experiences, many have written advice which they hope will be particularly helpful to other men. Again, if it resonates with other people, then I know they'll be over the moon. If you're a man and it doesn't resonate with you, I can only apologise. The last thing I want to do is to make people feel boxed in. For most people, there will be some ideas which resonate with them and some ideas which annoy them, making them scream 'I'm not like that!' That's just the inevitable result of grouping half the planet into a single homogenous group. I know that all men are different. I know that every reader has their own ways of processing feelings. When I work as a listener and mentor, I know that some advice resonates with some people, but annoys others. If something connects with you then make it work for you. If something doesn't, then move on for now, but consider coming back to it at a later date.

I've spoken to a wide range of men who have experienced feelings in different ways. This book includes the stories of some of these men who have found their own ways of managing emotions. These are stories of people who have learned ways to pull themselves together, with the support of others. Most of these ideas are more effective than distraction and other short-term strategies. Some of their stories may resonate with you, while others might not. This book is also the distilled experience of over thirty years of listening to men and boys talk about their feelings.

This book also touches on society's changing relationship with men. With such a huge topic, all I can do is talk to other men, as well as offer my own distorted perspective. Each voice offers up their perspective, so each voice is important. It's time to listen to men talk about their feelings. This is an important story to tell. This is a start of a conversation, a conversation which men need to start having about their feelings. And all of us have a duty to lean in a little closer to hear.

In this book, I'd love to provoke some thought and maybe offer some comfort. I'd also hope that people can find encouragement. Encouragement that they're not alone, that what they are going through is 'normal', that there is support out there, and that there is more than one way to pull yourself together.

What is the Project?

If a very wise person said that they had found the key to emotional health, what do you think they would say? There are many keys to emotional health, and I've included many in this book, but YOUR key to emotional health may not be the same as mine. We all build up unhealthy habits over time which can hold us back, and a large part of this project is understanding those, challenging them, tackling them, and replacing them with healthier habits.

The project involves many things, including:

- becoming self-reflective about your emotional health

- increasing your levels of average happiness

- managing your emotional health in a sustainable way

- implementing wellbeing tips which help you find a few more ups, and a few less downs

- building effective rhythms and healthy habits

- replacing unhelpful short term coping strategies, with more effective coping strategies.

How This Book Works

The book is written in short chapters which all end with a clearly defined key point. Everything about the book is designed to make it engaging and approachable. There is no jargon nor long explanations; instead there are true life experiences alongside very practical ideas. There are also lots of lists and top tips and case studies. This book explains clearly why talking about feelings is important, and gives some practical ideas on how to make this more achievable. It contains a system which I have developed over many years and use regularly with people. This system is designed as a simple, usable long-term project.

I'm using the phrase 'pull yourself together' to describe the long-term project of managing emotional health.

I have divided the project into sections to reflect the stages we go through when tackling a large project. We spend some time weighing up the idea first. Then we spend some time gaining a good understanding of what's involved, which I've called Part Two. In these first two sections of the book you will notice a lot of self-reflective questions. You may want to make notes, or simply pause and think about your own responses. This is the stage where you are learning your own rhythms and habits. As we move towards parts three and four, the project of managing your mental health will be fully underway, and the reflective questions give way to suggestions and practical ideas. Like any good project, preparation is everything, and the questions in parts one and two are important preparatory tools. The hard work of parts three and four will be made simpler because of the self-reflective thinking you will already have done.

Even when we are fully stuck into the project, around part four in this book, we will have days when we rest from it. We don't ever really rest from the project of improving our emotional health, but you will want days when you give your brain a break from focusing directly on it. Lastly, in part five, I focus on a few more keys to emotional health.

Many aspects of this book are designed to feel like a supportive friend. The different voices I have collected together, the conversations about emotional health, and the lists and anecdotes are all designed to make you feel like you are sitting with a supportive friend. The self-reflective questions in the first two parts of the book are the kind of things that a supportive friend or professional helper might ask. Some questions are light-hearted, while others are more hard-hitting. One of the roles of professional helpers is to ask poignant, reflective questions. Allowing yourself time and space to self-reflect is an important part of this project.

Don't rush these questions, try and get used to looking inward and being honest. Whether you write on these pages, or find a notebook, is up to you. The questions are designed to stimulate thought and self-reflection. There are no right answers, but honesty and openness will help you.

I've tended to categorise the project of improving your emotional health alongside fun, but challenging, projects so far, but for some men it might currently seem more like a blocked drain. There are sometimes challenging projects which we put off and put off because they are definitely not fun. But, like a blocked drain, ignoring it will only make it worse. There has to come a day when you roll up your sleeves and tackle it. The reality is that you are already embarking on the long-term project of pulling yourself together, by reading this book. You have already rolled up your sleeves. You have already taken the most important step – the first. You have moved through the stage most of us go through, of ignoring or denying your struggles, and now you are taking on a project. The amazing, challenging, transforming project of pulling yourself together, man.

PART ONE

DECIDING TO TAKE ON THE PROJECT

You know you love a project

You know you love a project, don't you? Something to focus on, something to sink your teeth into, something that gets you up in the morning with a spring in your step. Something to tinker on, something to distract you, something to while away the hours. I love a project.

My five favourite projects:

- Building a go-kart

- Inventing a board game

- Home brewing

- Building a gin bar

- Turning a wasteland into a beach garden.

All these projects have excited me and scared me. They have seemed daunting and impossible at times, but gradually they have seemed achievable. I remember building go-karts as a teenager. I would find some pram wheels and some old wood, and I would start making a plan, or throwing things together randomly depending on how I felt. Soon I'd encounter a problem which was beyond me. How does an axle work? How do I use this electric drill? I'd then do some additional research by reading around, or asking around, till I'd solved that problem. Or I'd get someone to physically help me. In this way, gradually the project would turn from something beyond me into something fun.

The project of improving your wellbeing may seem daunting at the start, and you may encounter challenges on the way. You may have to do some additional research, or even ask for help. I'd still encourage you to dive in and make a start. All the best projects seem daunting at first but if you work on them step by step you will always make progress.

The best kinds of project have their own mysterious language and strange complexities which only fanatics understand. I love this sense of entering a new world. When I first became interested in inventing board games, I found a whole group of people using words and phrases I'd never encountered before. I discovered that my tiny amount of knowledge was woefully inadequate. There are some phrases which can't be avoided, but they can be explained. It didn't take long before I was happily using these terms as well as anyone. The world of wellbeing and emotional health, which we enter in this book, might have some unusual phrases and ideas which could be useful to your understanding. I will explain these throughout, so try not to be put off by these phrases, and embrace them as part of your project.

To consider your usual rhythms and habits, we're going to spend some time considering how you usually approach a project. Consider a large, exciting, but daunting, project you have undertaken in the last few years. It could be anything: a DIY project, learning a language, raising money for a cause, learning a new skill, fixing something, setting yourself a resolution. As you answer these questions, start to consider if some of your ingrained habits and behaviours around how you tackle a project could provide some insights into your wellbeing habits. No need to over-think this at this early stage, but consider this next set of questions as a gentle introduction to self-reflection.

What was your project?

How did you decide on that project?

How did you start?

What was your first major challenge?

Did you ask for support when things got difficult?

Did you make any major mistakes?

When you made mistakes, how did you feel?

Did you finish?

In general, how did it go? Do you consider it a success? How are you measuring that? Think back on all the ups and downs. Remember the times you wanted to give up, but you pushed on through. Or maybe you didn't, and you stopped at the first hurdle. That's ok too. Reflecting on that experience will help you next time. It's not just successes which fuel us. By allowing yourself time to understand your rhythms and habits you have already made progress. Perhaps, as you answered the questions, it occurred to you that you put things off for a long time, and that this isn't always helpful. Or perhaps you dive in without adequate preparation. Perhaps you have a habit of giving up without asking for support. Perhaps you leave a lot of projects unfinished. Recognising habits which hold you back is an important first step in changing them.

In this book you are encouraged to build a healthy emotional approach to life as a project. This is the model I want to use as I encourage you to think about your wellbeing and emotional health. It is a pattern which has worked well for many people, particularly men.

> *What worries do you currently have about tackling your emotional health as a long-term project?*
>
> *Do you feel that you'll get enough support if you decide to tackle your emotional health?*

Managing emotional health is a long-term project. It's an ongoing work stretching sometime into the future. It will bring ups and downs. Sometimes it will make you get up in the morning with a spring in your step; other times you will have to push through the hard times. Sometimes you will need to reach out for help, and other times you will find your own breakthroughs. Like all the best projects, it will be worth it. In the end, it is the best project, and brings the best rewards.

KEY POINT: *One of the KEYS to managing emotional health is to approach it like a project.*

Failure?

Here is some good news: you can't fail when it comes to improving your wellbeing. By focusing on it, you have already made progress. The biggest enemy of wellbeing is ignoring or denying your emotional health. By the very fact that you have got this far in this book, you're already not doing that. If this was a race, you'd have already overtaken half the field. But good news is sometimes followed by bad news, and the bad news is that, although you can't fail, there will be setbacks. Improving emotional health is never linear. It's never a straight line. It's a series of ups and downs with moments of setback. Progress can be measured if you take a long-term view, but at particular points things will be getting worse before they can become better. There are reasons for this and they are to do with how the brain stores difficulties, how we build and dismantle habits, how some struggle can help us, and the purposes of difficult emotions: all things which will be covered in more depth. For now, understand that things will get better if you focus on your wellbeing but there will definitely be setbacks on the way. Look back at the project you explored above. Think particularly about the rhythms and habits you fell back on regarding the challenges and setbacks. Remember that 'failure' is the best teacher. No one with a big dream has ever achieved it without setbacks along the way. If you look at any 'successful' people, they will have a story to tell about their biggest 'failures'. It is these setbacks which help us build resilience, which is one of the most important tools you need for this project.

Five tools needed for this project:

- Resilience
- Openness
- Bravery
- Acceptance
- Support.

In my son's school they use the phrase: FAIL = First Attempt In Learning. Resilience is not something which comes easily to people who have not encountered huge setbacks. Resilience is a tool which only comes from bitter experience. Again, it is by focusing on, and gradually undoing, unhealthy habits that we make space to build healthier habits. So, let's consider your relationship to failure generally. Be honest. Remember, the more we fail, the quicker we build resilience. Failure can be a great teacher, so let's reflect on failure.

What emotions do you particularly associate with failure?

Write down three things you think you failed at that hurt.
1.
2.
3.

Write down three things you think you failed at, which don't bother you.

1.

2.

3.

Write down something you kept going at, despite setbacks.

Write down something which you stopped because of setbacks.

Write down something you'd like to try again at.

In general, consider your usual relationship to failure. Do you hate it, deny it, or do you learn from it? What helps you back on your feet? What emotions do you particularly associate with failure? Does it make you angry, depressed, or more determined? Recognising and understanding these habits is the first step to changing them.

> **KEY POINT:** *You can't fail when it comes to focusing on your wellbeing. By thinking about it, you are already improving it.*

A job well done

Something which makes a project so satisfying is the warm feeling of achievement. There is no feeling like it. It's one reason why people push themselves to tackle great things. It's why people spend rainy days in the garden or tinkering on a car. In addition to the satisfaction and reward of the task itself, there is the expectation of the future reward of sitting back and basking in the satisfaction of a job well done. All the short-term setbacks and challenges will be forgotten in that moment when the task is complete. It's one of the best feelings in the world.

Five things which are difficult but satisfying:

- Climbing a mountain

- Running a marathon

- Parenting a child

- Writing a book

- Learning a language.

My allotment is hard work. When I first got it, it was so overgrown that it took me three days of hacking down weeds before I discovered a hidden wheelbarrow in the overgrowth. I'll never win against the weeds and the slugs and the pests, but I'll have small victories on the way. Whenever I go to the allotment, I take a flask of tea, which I ignore while I battle away to the point of exhaustion. And only then do I sit on my blue chair and unscrew the lid of my flask and sit back with a feeling of complete contentment. That feeling can't be reached through short-cuts. That's what makes it so precious.

People think that they enjoy rest. But rest loses its sheen after a few days or a few weeks. Rest is most beautiful when it comes after hard work.

I've had times in my life when rest has been imposed on me, during times of illness and times of unemployment, and I don't remember those times fondly. Like many of us, I was surprised how much I struggled during lockdown. I thought I needed a rest when I was first put on furlough from work. But it wasn't long before I realised that I needed purpose as much as I needed rest. Lockdown during the pandemic was a collective cultural experience that we all went through, but our experiences differed wildly. This has made it harder to talk about. Instead of bringing us together in some collective experience, it has made the experiences of one group of people, those who were unable to work through lockdown, seem at odds with another group of people, those whose work increased. For me, one of the interesting things about lockdown was seeing how many people in the first group discovered that they didn't like rest as much as they expected to. I know countless people who thought they would enjoy the rest of furlough, but then found themselves aimless and dissatisfied. Purposelessness is disheartening. It can be bad for our self-esteem. One of the keys to managing emotional health is to find a balance between rest and purpose. Keeping these two opposing forces in a balance that suits the individual is not as easy as it sounds. At times our need for purpose pushes us too far and we need to rest; at other times we become over-rested and lose purpose. These rhythms change constantly throughout our life. Humans are seasonal: we have times when we have seemingly endless energy to push forward purposely, and other times when we need to retreat and rest.

In this next section of questions you will be asked to think about your relationship to purpose and rest. There are no right answers, but, as with other self-reflective questions, think about habits which hold you back and habits which drive you forward.

Do you consider yourself to be ambitious?

What drives you on?

Are you good at recognising when you need to rest?

What helps you rest?

Finding purpose can help us to find wellbeing. It is great to wake up with a sense of energy and purpose. But we can also lose ourselves in this purpose, and become so hard-driven that we don't take time to enjoy things. Finding an ongoing sustainable rhythm which balances effort and rest is one of the keys to wellbeing. It rarely happens by accident. It takes thought and self-reflection to achieve this. It's an on-going balancing act, which is constantly changing. Imagine yourself on a tightrope and someone is pulling your balancing bar one way, and someone else is shaking the rope. That can be how finding a balance between purpose and rest can feel. But the more often we reflect on it, and the more we constantly adjust, the more chance we have of finding success.

Right now, do you feel like you need more purpose in your life?

Write down four things which help you find purpose:

1.

2.

3.

4.

Right now, do you feel like you need more rest in your life?

Write down four things which help you find rest:

1.

2.

3.

4.

In general, how good are you at balancing purpose and rest in your life?

To renew your emotional health is a project which will sometimes involve un-doing ingrained thought patterns. It will almost certainly demand some changes in your habits of behaviour and thought. Changing ingrained behaviours takes hard work. Change takes place slowly and with support. Sometimes it demands effort, but sometimes it demands rest. Finding the right balance is key.

KEY POINT: *One of the KEYS to managing emotional health is to find a balance between rest and purpose.*

Do I love running?

I go running a couple of times a week. I'm not particularly fast, and I can't run particularly far, but I am better than I was two years ago when I first laced up my trainers. One day I was getting ready to head out for a run in the rain at the same time as trying to convince my daughter to do her homework. I told her that if I could go running in the rain then she could spend half an hour doing homework.

'That's not the same at all,' she protested. 'You love running.'

And I stood there asking myself a question I'd never thought about. Do I love running? And I'm pretty sure that I don't. There is always a part of me that hates it. It's hard, repetitive work, and it makes my lungs burst and my legs ache. But I love stopping. And I love the feeling of satisfaction I get from a job well done. And I like getting slightly better at it over time. And I love the energy it gives me, and the feeling of wellbeing. And I have to keep these things in mind, because if I focus on how hard it is, I'll just give up. If I focus on the things which I do love, then I'll keep going.

The commitment and community and the connection to nature it brings are all really good for my emotional health. I've also been more in touch with my own body. I've noticed my breathing and learnt how to control it slightly better. And after an early run the rest of the day seems so much more manageable.

These concepts are also helpful for managing emotional health. It can take commitment, community, and connection, as well as an understanding of your own body.

I asked some male friends the question, 'what do you do which is hard, but satisfying?' Here are some responses.

Things men do which are hard, but satisfying

- Weights

- Running

- Gardening

- Going to work

- Staying married

- Playing a musical instrument

- Parenting

- Pursuing a dream

- Losing weight

- Listening to people

- Cleaning

- Putting up Christmas decorations

- Not drinking

- Public speaking

- Apologising

I love the breadth of these answers. I asked people separately, so they didn't hear each other's answers, and I just love the honesty shown here. There's a humour in some answers, a raw honesty in others, and a wounded heart in others.

Write down three things that do you do regularly which are hard, but satisfying:

1.

2.

3.

When I help people manage their emotional health, and people embark on the project of improving their wellbeing, as you are doing here, there is eventually a conversation about Recovery Pastimes. Most people who find healthier thinking habits also find it useful to develop hobbies, pastimes and projects which help improve their wellbeing. These will be explored in greater depth in Part Three. Sometimes the things which become Recovery Pastimes are the things you least expect to. I never expected running to help with my emotional wellbeing, but it definitely does.

KEY POINT: *Difficult but satisfying things can be good for your emotional health.*

Why do some men struggle when talking about feelings?

Many things can help people with their emotional health, but nothing is a substitute for talking. My experience is that, in the main, men are less practised at talking about their feelings than women. It doesn't always come naturally. Men often respond badly to being 'forced' to talk about their feelings. In the right circumstances, with the right friends, in just the right moment, most men I know actually love to open up. Sometimes, you have to catch people in just the right moment.

I asked some friends of mine why they think that some men struggle to talk about feelings. Here are their responses.

Why do some men struggle to talk about feelings?

- I think that the reason men do not want to talk about issues is that to do so would be to admit to a sense of failure in their role as 'head of the house'.

- Because of perceived roles of men – as portrayed in the media/wider society.

- The problem is who to talk to! Doctors have no time to be 'listeners' and I don't think that many men have close 'confidants'.

- Because of the role models that brought us up.

- Sometimes I find it hard to put feelings into words.

- Because it's not modelled to them by fathers or any other male role models.

- It's a sign of weakness, and 'real' men shouldn't be weak.

- People might just laugh.

- It never seems to be the 'right time' to be vulnerable.

- It's been identified as a 'woman's thing'.

- It's 'easier' not to.

I love these answers, but they also make me sad. There is no reason anyone should feel these things. Most of these things are false misconceptions which have become ingrained over time. I have often opened up about deep feelings, and no one has ever laughed. As far as I know, no one has thought me weak because I've shared my feelings. You might think these things are changing, and maybe they are, but the associated hurts take a long time to heal. These comments were all collected in the last two years, which tells me that, even now, many men are being held back by these thoughts on sharing their feelings.

> *When did you last open up about your feelings?*

> *Did you get the response that you expected?*

> *How did you feel afterwards?*

I spend a lot of time listening to people talk; it's a big part of my job. These listening sessions are not the same as opening up to your mates in a pub, but there are things we can learn from them. Everyone is different but there are some common tropes in listening sessions. There are some who approach a listening session as an 'open book'. As soon as someone offers to listen, they willingly and gratefully pour out their lives. They tell their stories and talk about their feelings, and openly admit to their struggles. My experience, and the experience of my colleagues, is that these 'open books' are rarely male. There are some men who approach a listening session like this, but they are rare. Some men take weeks getting to this point, and some never get there at all. Some get there intermittently, and for some there is a personal cost to opening up. Some have covered themselves in way too much armour, some are suspicious of opening up, and some don't know how to. One of the reasons men are so unpractised at talking about themselves is that they don't always know how. Men are spectacularly good at denying problems. Men have a tradition of hiding their head in the sand over things: not visiting doctors, denying when they've got problems and not admitting they need help. They are just not used to talking about problems or feelings. The language of feelings seems uncomfortable, or feminine, or inadequate. Some men have grown up with little freedom to talk about their feelings. Or, even if they have, the response has often been unhelpful.

Would you describe yourself as an open book when it comes to talking about feelings?

A common response to talking about feelings with men I know is a 'shields up' response. I see this in my listening sessions too. Someone might sit with their arms folded, a closed expression on their face, unwilling to let down their guard. They have covered their hurts with layer upon layer of armour, which seems too risky to dismantle. They might not even know how to dismantle it and let someone in. One of the reasons why men can be bad at talking about feelings is that they have learnt to hide their feelings. When I listen to women talk, they often see their problems as something outside of themselves that they can have help in fixing. Whereas, when I listen to men talk, they are more likely to see themselves as the problem, and therefore equate the offer of help with implied criticism.

> *Do you recognise yourself in this*
> *description, putting up defences?*

Another possible response is that of the 'quick fix'. A typical male response to problems is to expect answers. Why should feelings be any different? What's the best and quickest way to fix difficult feelings. Sadly, 'fix' in this example usually means hide, or distract. The person who is after a quick fix is much more likely to find a new distraction, or way of masking feelings which don't go away, and simply store up problems for another time. One of the reasons why men can be bad at talking about feelings is that they are looking for simple answers and are unwilling to confront more serious issues.

> *Do you recognise yourself in this*
> *description, wanting a quick-fix,*
> *or nothing?*

Let's think of a real individual. I have changed the name, but this is a real example of someone we can look at as a case study.

CASE STUDY: **JOSIAH**

I am sitting in a room in a mainstream school, which is used as a listening room. I see students for half an hour to talk about their feelings. As one student leaves, another walks in. He sits at the offered chair but doesn't get comfortable. He sits forward on the chair and keeps his bag on his knee, building a small barrier. In an ideal world, I would know his name and why he's been sent to me, but the busyness of schools means that doesn't always happen. I have to ask his name, which he tells me is Josiah. After explaining who I am, I ask him who has sent him and he tells me that the pastoral year head has sent him. This means that there is probably an issue at home or school. But I am still none the wiser, so I ask why he thinks he's been sent to me. A question which is, probably deservedly, met with a shoulder shrug. After some fishing for answers I know all sorts of things about him. Things about his family and school life, and friends and hobbies. I even know a bit about his feelings, which he talks about reluctantly, as if I'm asking about the dark side of the moon. He talks about feelings as if he's talking about something which is beyond any human understanding. He's not rude, or unpleasant, but he gives the impression that there has been some kind of mistake. Twenty-nine minutes into the session he is already on his feet and on his way to the door. Whilst in the doorway he turns around as if to say goodbye, and tells me that his mum died two days ago.

Why do you think Josiah didn't mention his mother's death straight away?

Why do you think he mentioned it just as he was leaving?

One of the reasons why men can be unpractised at talking about feelings is that they are afraid. It's not uncommon for people in listening sessions to hold back a vital truth until the last possible minute, where they then have the cover of walking away. This phenomenon is known among listeners as the 'doorway disclosure'. This type of response can be common in arguments as well. It is not unusual for a man to talk and talk but then fire out the most important detail right at the last minute before storming off. There is a fragility to these responses. The person needs help. They desperately want someone to understand them, but they are also scared. They throw out their greatest need almost as a hand-grenade before running for cover.

> *Do you recognise the habit of 'doorway disclosure' in your own life, perhaps in how you approach arguments?*

> *Would you describe yourself as afraid to talk about feelings?*

Some people seem angry. They may open up one week and close themselves down another week. They may let you in a little and then slam the door. Often, these people are seen as angry, but there's something deeper going on. People have frequently misinterpreted their strong feelings as anger. One of the reasons why men can be bad at talking about feelings is that people misinterpret their strong feelings as anger.

> *Do you often get told that you are angry?*

> *Do you often feel that the description is inaccurate?*

How do you feel when people call you angry,
but you feel there is more going on?

It's not just anger that gets misinterpreted by other people. People are often terrible at interpreting strong male emotions. The reality is that society currently has an ambivalent and difficult relationship with strong male feelings. Which creates suspicion. Perhaps the most common male response on first encountering a listener is suspicion. Not about anything dark or mysterious, just the learnt suspicion of having been misunderstood before.

One of the reasons why men can be bad at talking about feelings is that they are suspicious of being misunderstood.

When you talk about feelings,
are you more:

- Open book

- Shields up

- Quick fix

- Afraid

- Angry

- Suspicious?

None of these responses is wrong, but some can be more helpful than others. As a listener, I'd love it if all the people who came to me were an open book. It would make my life easier, but, more than that, it is a generally healthy response. All the science suggests that talking about feelings does help. It's not easy for a lot of men to talk about their feelings in the first place. But then I look at culture and wonder if we've somehow made things even harder. In the end, when everything else has been stripped away I think that most men would LOVE to understand their feelings and talk about them more. Granted, there is a lot of stripping away to be done, and some serious soul-searching to be done as a society. If talking helps, which it undoubtedly does, then people need to find ways to make it easier for everyone. So, perhaps the question shouldn't be 'why are men so bad at talking about their feelings?' but 'why are people so bad at helping men talk about their feelings?'

When I trained as a listener, I was told that the best opening question was, 'what would you like to talk about today?' This question can work with open book types, but it is way too subtle for some men. I had to work hard to find new ways to help men open up about their feelings. There are no perfect opening questions, but my experience is that some opening questions work better for some types of people than others.

- The 'shields up' character can sometimes respond to: 'tell me about some things which make you happy', followed later by 'tell me about some things which frustrate you.'

- The 'quick fix' character might respond to: 'what's your biggest challenge right now?'

- The 'afraid' character might respond to: 'if you had a magic wand to fix one issue in your life, what would it be?'

- The 'angry' character might respond to: 'do you get enough support in your life?'

- The 'suspicious' character might respond to: 'what do people keep doing that you dislike, and what do you wish they would change?'

These are only suggestions, and there are many other great questions which help people to open up.

> **KEY POINT:** *Talking about feelings does help, so people need to find ways to make this easier.*

Fancy a coffee?

In the end it's not always about the question, but the setting. Think of times in your life where you have found it easiest to talk about feelings. You probably won't remember what you were asked, but you will probably remember the setting.

Which setting would best help you open up?

- On a camping trip
- Staring at a bonfire
- Whilst supping a real ale
- On a long hike
- In a coffee shop
- By a lake
- On a lads' weekend away
- Sitting comfortably by a real fire
- On a beach
- After climbing a hill.

> **KEY POINT:** *Think about a setting which would encourage you to open up*

Where have all the feelings gone?

Like a lot of men, I used to experience incredibly strong emotions growing up and into my teenage years. When I was a child, I was often described as highly-strung. People didn't mean it as a compliment. They meant that I was always wound so tight that I might snap at any moment. Then I was described as an angsty teenager. Teenage boys these days are more likely to be described as snowflakes. People sometimes talk about males with strong emotions as if there is something wrong with them. They might label them with negative terms, and when they have strong feelings people ask what's wrong, giving the impression that strong feelings are wrong.

Popular insults for men with strong feelings

- Man up
- Boys don't cry
- You're such a girl
- Grow a pair
- Crazy
- Highly-strung
- Snowflake
- Pull yourself together, man!

Something dulled my feelings in my twenties and thirties. I may have done it myself. I wasn't fully aware of the change at the time because it crept up slowly. But this new dullness took hold. In the end, it was becoming a dad which re-awoke incredibly strong emotions. When I held my first-born child, I felt a rush of strong emotions which I didn't even know that I'd lost. And I loved it. It was like coming home.

CASE STUDY: **CALLUM**

I have been working with a teenage boy for three weeks. He is a school refuser and finds school difficult, but can't explain why. I've got lots of notes from other helpers who have found that he just can't turn his feelings into words. This has also been my experience. He doesn't say much about anything, and it's hard to make sense of him as an individual. I'm not even sure of his likes and dislikes. I just know that he hates school. He struggles to talk about anything, but as soon as he gets close to talking about feelings he's even more distressed. A noticeable change comes over him. He starts to shake and clam up, and struggles to speak at all. At the end of week three I ask him to try and catalogue his feelings on his phone as simple notes, to try and keep some track of the highs and lows of his week. The next week he gets his phone out and reads his notes. He hardly draws breath and talks solidly for five minutes straight. As he speaks, I make notes, trying to summarise his feelings. I write quickly, trying to keep up with him. All I'm trying to do is to summarise his feelings. I'm not making any observations, I'm just cataloguing these strong feelings that have been bubbling away inside him. When he stops, I have three solid sides of A4 laying bare the overwhelming and extraordinary feelings of an amazing person.

Why do you think Callum struggled to turn his feelings into words?

Why was Callum able to catalogue his feelings on his phone?

I love my strong emotions. I would encourage everyone to seek out the experiences which re-awaken strong feelings, especially if they have become dulled over time. If I cry openly, people tell me that I'm in touch with my feminine side. So I have to explain to them that that's my masculine side. That's the side which got re-awoken by fatherhood. Not everyone has this same experience, but I'd love it if people found ways to open the floodgates to strong emotions.

I asked a friend, 'when have you experienced difficult emotions?'

When my daughter plays the piano, I could sit and listen to her for hours. I can't truly put my finger on why, but if I speculate it could be that I was musical myself when I was young, and the music was my only real social outlet. I recognise how much practice and effort goes into being able to play well, but I also recognise the positive social impact it will have on her life. I can also see that she clearly does it because she enjoys it, not because she is told to. When she plays something I put my hand on my chest like a flippin' American president (!) and really 'feel' it! (If I could put a raised eyebrow emoji here I would, because it still surprises me that I feel so strongly about this!)

Here are several other responses.

When have you experienced overwhelming emotions?

- Childbirth

- Watching Torquay United

- My dog dying

- On discovering that I had been betrayed

- Lewis Hamilton's first world championship

- During and following an extended period of verbal and physical bullying at school, leading to speech impediment, social anxiety and genuine fear of being singled out in class etc.

- Reading books to my children

- On being forced out of my family (matrimonial) home

- When my niece died

- When my wife had an affair, left me, took virtually everything we owned and, most importantly, removed my children from my care

- When flying at 30,000 feet with a couple of glasses of red wine I can find myself getting completely emotional at the most uninspiring and bland movies – which would not move me if I were on the ground!

- Road rage

- Following bad leakage in new house, any unexpected sounds my heart would race and I would be overwhelmed with anxiety… only intentional controlled breathing and prayer seemed to calm me

- At Glastonbury, watching Radiohead.

These responses are a mix of the extreme highs and lows of life. They are also a snapshot of many different emotions. Each phrase taken individually could probably be broken down into a whole series of different emotions. Take childbirth. We can imagine the emotional roller-coaster of hope, fear, anxiety, confusion, exhilaration, and elation playing on a loop, and we'll still get nowhere close to describing the full experience.

> *When have you experienced overwhelming emotions?*
>
> *What were some of the key emotions in this experience?*
>
> *Try asking a friend, when have you experienced overwhelming emotions?*

As an emotional health specialist, I never talk about wrong feelings, or bad feelings. Some feelings are more difficult than others, but that doesn't make them wrong. But people still fear these difficult emotions. And rightly so, sometimes. Difficult emotions are hard work. They can blind-side you when you least expect it. They can sit heavily on your shoulders. They can impact your everyday life. One of the respondents continues,

> *The emotions were so great I found myself breaking down and crying on numerous occasions. I think the feeling can probably be summed up in two words, 'loss' and 'helplessness' – not at the betrayal, but more about everything you have worked for and the future you planned, and none of those options are on the table any longer – future options become much 'smaller'.*

Faced by this heartbreak it can seem wiser to distract yourself from strong feelings, avoiding them or ignoring them. It can seem more sensible to keep strong feelings dulled down. It's not. The truth is that they are still there either way. Hiding from difficult feelings doesn't make them go away. That's not how it works. Difficult emotions impact on your body and in your life, whether you acknowledge them or not. In the long run it is safer and healthier to acknowledge them than to hide or deny them.

> **KEY POINT:** *It is good to acknowledge strong feelings.*

The man drawer in the brain

I've got a man-drawer in my house. It drives my wife mad. All the random things which will be useful one day get shoved in there. There they sit all higgledy-piggledy until one day I need something which I know must be in there somewhere. Inevitably I can't find it, so, after a frustrating hour of digging around among old batteries and dried up glue, I give up and buy a new one. A man drawer should be useful and yet it isn't. We all know this, but we all still have one. It's how we are wired.

Ten items in people's man drawers

- Dead batteries
- Charging leads for lost phones
- Foreign coins
- Dead phones
- Instructions for old appliances
- Takeaway menus
- Fuses
- Wire

- Golf balls (even though you don't play golf)
- Car keys for your old car

Few, if any, of these things are useful. Even the takeaway menus never get looked at now my wife orders everything online. And yet the drawer is still there, taking up prime space in my house.

Write down three things in your man drawer:
1.
2.
3.

Man drawers are full of clutter. If you do want something, the amount of clutter makes it hard to find anyway. I hate to tell you that, worse than this, is the man drawer in your brain. At some point almost every male that has ever lived learns to shove difficult emotions and unwanted feelings into a closed drawer in their brain. There they sit gathering dust but never really going anywhere. Sadly, though, they do impact your life. Our brains and bodies are not two separate things. They are completely connected, and what is shoved away in the drawer in your brain will spill into your body and affect you.

Or, worse still, one day the drawer gets too full, the bottom falls out and these things spill out all over your life. There isn't a way around this. It's just like the man drawer in your house. One day, you have to roll up your sleeves and tackle it head on: which, by the very fact that you are reading this book, is what you are already doing!

> **KEY POINT:** *Most people hide difficult feelings away, but it is important to acknowledge them.*

The myth of Neanderthals

The idea of man as an emotional Neanderthal, with a narrow emotional range, is a persistent one. People perpetuate this myth in various ways. When do we ever see media representations of men with wide-ranging complicated emotional worlds? When do we ever read about them, or even talk about them? I once heard a neighbour describe her husband to my wife as 'a typical male, he doesn't do feelings'. Everything about this description upsets me. From the word typical, through to the fact that he does do feelings, she's just not recognising them. The myth of the emotional Neanderthal is everywhere in our society. And the trouble is that it is really damaging. Listen to these words from a married man in his forties, when asked what he wanted people to understand about his emotional health.

> *I wish people would see me as a fully functioning human being. I might not express emotions the same as them, but that doesn't mean that I don't have them. The other day I was struggling with anxiety when I was out with my family. I guess I'd gone a bit quiet and withdrawn, but I was thinking about some things. When my eldest*

daughter asked my wife what was up, she said, 'Dad's just angry.' I tried to explain that I wasn't angry, because I hadn't been, but the more I protested the angrier I sounded! And then the word 'just' started bugging me and I probably did become angry! I was frustrated because all my complicated feelings had been dismissed with one word. And I don't really want my girls growing up and doing the same thing when they are older. This kind of thing happens all the time, and all of us seem powerless to stop it.

This man can recognise his feelings. He knows that he's feeling anxious, but he's feeling boxed in when other people don't see that. If people were less quick to pigeonhole his feelings, he'd have more freedom to express them. We need to have a culture shift in how we talk about men and feelings. It's not ok to keep perpetuating the myth of the Neanderthal. People often talk about how their father's generation struggled to express their feelings. But the reasons for this are complicated and multi-faceted.

What do you want people to understand about your emotional health?

- Tough question... don't think I've ever really thought this through... perhaps that I'm not as 'together' as they think I am, to be kind, and to let me know if I've offended them too as that would upset me not knowing.

- That I don't always understand it! But that I'd welcome questions. I think questions help us make sense of things, so people can always just ask.

These responses talk about what other people think and how it impacts them. It seems time to move past the myth of the emotional Neanderthal. Change doesn't primarily need to come about in how men express their feelings; it needs to come about in how other people hear them. Feelings get expressed. They can be loud or subtle, but they come out somewhere. When men express feelings in different ways than people expect, then society needs to become better at hearing this.

> **KEY POINT:** *There are no Neanderthals; all of us experience emotions.*

How to be a man

My wife first became pregnant at a time when my dad was a missing person. These two things coming together overwhelmed me. Needing people to talk to, I searched for a group where I could discuss these things with other men and found nowhere where I could discuss my hopes and fears. I didn't know how to be a dad. As I struggled with this problem it seemed to grow. Did I even know how to be a man? Luckily, this situation has changed. On a personal level, my dad came home and continues to be a great dad. And on a societal level, there are now groups set up for men to talk.

I sometimes feel that I am the least manly man on the planet. When I first met my wife, before we were married, we had a date in the Science Museum. They had a computer programme that was supposed to work out from your responses if you were male or female. It was supposed to be pretty accurate, but it thought I was a woman. Which didn't surprise my wife one little bit! A few years later we did a marriage course. The advice for males didn't make any sense to me, and the advice to females didn't make any sense to my wife. Things were fine as long as I took the advice for ladies, and she took the advice for men. Not that she's manly: she's not; and not that I'm effeminate: I'm not, I just don't fit the male stereotype.

Perhaps none of us do. I do find male stereotypes frustrating. They seem belittling and restrictive. They seem to be played out regularly. When I queue in the supermarket behind male and female couples, there is a common pantomime which takes place, and everyone knows their part. The wife takes control of the packing while the husband gets gently mocked for putting items in the wrong places.

Stereotypes are inevitable. In many ways they are just a short-cut to familiarity. They can be a way for people to bond quickly. In the supermarket the wife is bonding with the cashier through a shared experience.

But stereotypes can also be destructive. They push people towards identities which restrict them. They limit people's sense of choice and freedom. They create prejudices and can lead to discrimination.

What annoys you about male stereotypes?

- That they are so ingrained. That men have to have a lot of self-confidence before fighting these stereotypes.

- The stereotype which says that a man is either a hard-nut or a wimp.

- They make me feel like I don't fit in.

- They stopped me from discovering a lot of things I liked until later in life, when I was too old to care what people thought of me.

- The actual stereotype itself.

- I might have chosen art GCSE if it wasn't 'gay' for lads to do it when I was at school.

- It generally pigeonholes men, limiting options and ability to express themselves.

- Rugby! I don't understand it.

- The number of times I have been asked why I am no longer with the mother of my children, and by default not with my children... when asked this question you can hear the tone, see the body language, and you know you have already been judged. What did you do? Why are you not with them? The stereotype itself is shocking really – a no-win situation – man must be guilty.

- That we're all meant to like football.

- It's assumed I don't change nappies, do most of the cooking, house-work etc. – so patronising!

- When you see a man on TV these days you know he's either shown as a terrible person straight away, or, if not, he'll have some terrible dark secret. He's never actually good these days.

- They're always shown to look so macho.

Not all male stereotypes are destructive, but some are. And stereotypes hold people back. When men are struggling and they don't know how to reach out for help, then some of the blame needs to fall on the stereotypes and the people who perpetuate them. When the phrases we use are part of the problem then these need to be confronted head on. It is never ok to equate feelings with femininity. It is never ok to tell someone to man-up.

> **KEY POINT:** *Consider if you are hiding your true feelings because of stereotypes.*

Are you a wimp?

Some men have grown up with little freedom to talk about their feelings. Or they have encountered unhelpful responses. If someone isn't used to talking about problems, or feelings, how can they become more used to it? And, perhaps more importantly, how can people talk in a language of feelings which is just as relevant to men?

Feelings aren't masculine or feminine. Feelings are everyone's birth-right. And if people are being denied, or denying themselves, that birth-right, then something is wrong. We need to learn to democratise feelings. People need to find ways to help men talk about their feelings.

There is a recognised phenomenon where men sometimes see women as either angel or whore. This is sometimes called the Madonna-Whore dichotomy. These two extremes are seen as polar opposites. It doesn't allow people the freedom to be themselves, because they get polarised as one thing or another. Men with these ideas struggle to see women as both nurturing and sexual. They subconsciously see these two roles as mutually exclusive. These views are damaging for females, but they can be damaging for males as well. Males, who have imbibed these views, develop reductive, simplistic and critical ideas of women. Women can also develop these views as internalised oppression.

The Madonna-whore dichotomy damages society and damages female freedoms and male choices. The most common male equivalent is the Caveman-Wimp dichotomy. Many people polarise men's choices to the extremes of caveman or wimp. Over time these two things become seen as mutually exclusive. People act like you can be one or another, but not both, but this isn't true. Everyone has elements of both in them, or neither. This dichotomy is particularly damaging because one of the characteristics of the caveman is that he hides his feelings. Although some men fear the characterisation of the caveman, they are more scared of the characterisation of the wimp. Very few men take any esteem from the wimp characterisation. Men become so fearful of the wimp characterisation that the caveman, despite his obvious flaws, seems like the better choice.

Of course, the reality is much more complex, and men's choices are so much richer than this, but, if society only allows these two options, then people's freedoms get restricted. These viewpoints damage society as a whole. They damage relationships, families and society, as well as individual men.

> **KEY POINT:** *Despite what society says, there are infinite choices beyond Caveman or Wimp.*

Power made perfect in weakness

One of the ideas which I find helpful is to consider assertiveness. People are sometimes characterised as:

- Submissive

- Aggressive

- Assertive.

Submissive behaviour can stem from an assumption that your wants and needs are less important than others. Aggressive behaviour can stem from an assumption that your wants and needs are more important than others. Assertive behaviour can stem from an understanding that your wants and needs are important, as are the wants and needs of others. Not many people are naturally assertive. Sometimes people can build up behaviour patterns which are aggressive; sometimes they lean towards submission; but it is rare to meet people who are naturally assertive.

> *Often people's 'weaknesses' turn out to also be their strengths. Can you think of an example for you?*

> *Can you think of a time when you've expressed power through 'weakness'?*

Behaviour patterns can be changed. Assertive behaviour can be much more effective than other behaviour patterns. It is a way of approaching people and situations which clearly outlines your own wants and needs without conflicting with others. We can say no to things without feeling guilty, because we are able to communicate our own feelings.

We can assert ourselves when the occasion demands it, but happily choose not to when it's not necessary.

It can take some practice, but it is a good habit to develop.

To become assertive, it can be useful to:

- know exactly what you want

- be sure it is fair

- ask for it clearly

- stay calm

- accept both praise and criticism.

Think of the most assertive people you know. Consider how they communicate, consider how they handle conflict, consider how they act and behave. I think of the Knights of the Round Table when I think of assertiveness. They were powerful people who used their power to challenge injustice. They used their power for good.

I am not naturally assertive, but I have found that practising assertive behaviour has been helpful in managing my emotional health. By practising assertiveness, I can avoid some of the guilt of my submissive instincts and some of the anger of my aggressive instincts.

> **KEY POINT:** *Practising assertive behaviour can help people manage their emotional health.*

What's wrong with feelings?

When I first sat down to answer the question, what's wrong with feelings? my answer was going to be – nothing. Nothing is wrong with feelings. Then I worried that my simple answer was insulting. If there is nothing wrong with feelings, then why should anyone ignore them. There are times when we need a break from difficult feelings. We can still acknowledge them, and respond to them, but we also need a short break.

Five things to try when you're feeling down

- Start planning a new club to join, and do it
- Do a random act of kindness
- Learn something new
- Write down three things you are grateful for
- Talk about it.
- Feelings aren't bad or wrong, but they can be difficult. They can be difficult for various reasons:
  - *They hurt*
  - *They're confusing*
  - *They scare people away*
  - *They can feel overwhelming*
  - *They push people away*
  - *They can be misinterpreted.*

They can be all of these things and more. But then I think about men I know who haven't acknowledged their difficult feelings and hide away behind unhelpful habits.

Five Creative ways to feel good

- Write a letter (yes, an actual letter!)
- Carry around a doodle pad (doodling is good)
- Adult colouring (you never know)
- Learn to cook something new
- Learn to play an instrument.

I think of men I know who have turned to drink, or drugs, or pornography to push difficult feelings away, and I know that, although difficult emotions can be painful, it is more painful and destructive to ignore them.

> **KEY POINT:** *Difficult feelings can be painful but ignoring or hiding from them is destructive.*

You are the expert

You are the best expert there is on you. Regardless of how many years someone has studied you, they can't climb into your head and understand you completely. You are always going to be the best expert on you and your own brain, and even you will sometimes get things wrong. People's emotions are so complicated and elusive and indescribable that you will sometimes have to try things out as you learn to understand your own emotional world. If you feel like something definitely isn't for you, then it probably isn't; trust your own instincts – you know you better than I do!

Name some specific areas of your life which could do with more emotional health.

As you have been focusing on your emotional health, have you become better at noticing difficult feelings?

It's good to get help with dealing with difficult emotions, both through this book and talking to people. Get as much help as you can, but be prepared for times when this book and the experts say one thing and you think you know better. Sometimes you'll be right. There might also be times when this book and the experts say one thing and you think you know better, and you are wrong. There also might be times when this book and the experts say one thing and you agree with us and we're all wrong.

Five ways to feel less stressed

1. Read a good book

2. Watch something that makes you laugh

3. Tidy your wardrobe

4. Take a walk in a forest

5. Sit down somewhere comfy and remember a great day.

Between this book and people you've found to talk to and your own expertise of your own head, you'll hopefully get it right a few times and you'll grow in your understanding of your amazing emotional world. So, let's press on with our long-term project, of improving our wellbeing and managing our emotional health.

> **KEY POINT:** *Try to trust your instincts as you try out new ideas.*

PART TWO

UNDERSTANDING
THE PROJECT

The goal

Consider for a moment what good emotional health would look like for you. Before beginning a project, it is useful to have an idea of the end point. If you are going to invest time renewing and managing your emotional health, it is useful to consider what you are hoping for. What is the goal? Remember, a key part of the project will be recognising unhelpful habits, to gradually replace them with healthier ones. Think back to some of the things we have looked at so far.

As we have read about unhelpful habits, which ones have resonated with you?

Have you recognised any other unhealthy habits in your life which impact your well-being?

It could be useful to start thinking of the targets you are working towards as you tackle the project of your own emotional health. Of course, you are much too complex to be reduced to this one thing, but we are just trying to narrow down your targets.

The definition of emotional health

> *A person with good emotional health can express all emotions appropriately, and can maintain a balance of emotions so that difficult emotions are not dominant.*

This phrase sums up a key part of the project. This is what we are all aiming for. This is our collective goal. We might not reach it completely, but we can edge closer. Like all the best instructions, it is useful to gain a complete understanding of it before we begin. (Please feel free to insert the male stereotype of making the flat-pack furniture without the instructions here!) We are going to try and fully understand this template by breaking it into small steps. Let's look at some words and phrases.

'Can express'

> *'CAN EXPRESS' (A person with good emotional health **can express** all emotions appropriately, and can maintain a balance of emotions so that difficult emotions are not dominant.)*

How well can you express your emotions? Who do you express them to? How often do you express them? Denying, hiding or ignoring difficult emotions can be a good short-term strategy but it is a terrible long-term strategy. Hiding away feelings in the man drawer is not healthy or beneficial in the long term. A much healthier habit to build is that of clearly and regularly expressing emotions. This might involve stepping out of your comfort zones, or dismantling ingrained habits, but in the end it should lead to good emotional health.

> **KEY POINT:** *Learning to express emotions is good for you.*

'All emotions'

> *'ALL EMOTIONS' (A person with good emotional health can express **all emotions** appropriately, and can maintain a balance of emotions so that difficult emotions are not dominant.)*

Emotions can be difficult to understand. There is no consensus on how many core emotions humans have. Various different theories have been put forward. Theorists have variously listed core emotions as:

- Anger, disgust, fear, joy, sadness, surprise (Ekman, Friesen and Ellsworth)

- Desire, happiness, interest, surprise, wonder, sorrow (Frijda)

- Rage, terror, anxiety, joy (Gray)

- Fear, grief, love, rage (James)

- Anger, joy, sadness, fear, love, dislike, fondness (Lichi)

- Pain, pleasure (Mowrer)

- Happiness, sadness (Weiner and Graham).

These different theories only go to show how little we understand our emotions. Maybe it's always going to be impossible to get anywhere close to understanding what other people are feeling. The important thing to realise about emotions is that they are real. Scientists may not agree on our core emotions, but they agree on this. They are real, they are not some vague ethereal thing. They are actual chemical and hormonal reactions in your brain. They have a certain reality. The chemical and hormonal reactions have an effect, whether you acknowledge them or not. And although theorists disagree about core human emotions, humans have shown a vast talent for wide-ranging emotions. There is an infinite richness of things we can feel as human beings. If you have built up the habit of talking about your emotions as if they flit between anger and happiness, then you are not helping others to see the rich variety of things that you can feel. Start using a wider range of words to describe your emotions. As you start to explore your own emotions in this next section, try to think in broader terms than simply happiness and sadness.

What is your favourite emotion?

Write down three other words to describe this feeling:
1.
2.
3.

What is your least favourite emotion?

Write down three other words to describe this feeling:

1.

2.

3.

What is an emotion which you have ambivalent feelings towards, seeing both the positives and negatives?

What is an emotion you have heard other people talking about, but you rarely experience?

Emotions are complicated, but they don't have to be feared. A rich emotional world is your birth right. It may be that you have to understand your own emotions before other people have a chance to understand your emotions.

KEY POINT: *There is an infinite richness of things we can feel as human beings.*

'Appropriately'

> 'APPROPRIATELY' (A person with good emotional health can express all emotions **appropriately**, and can maintain a balance of emotions so that difficult emotions are not dominant.)

I could list a thousand inappropriate ways to express difficult emotions. These can include violence, reliance on pornography, infidelity, alcoholism, drug-taking, comfort-eating, running away. In the end they all have something in common: they all end up hurting the person or those around them. Often, destructive behaviours and habits are the result of feelings which have been hidden away.

> **KEY POINT:** Destructive behaviours are often the result of unresolved or unacknowledged feelings.

'Can maintain'

> 'CAN MAINTAIN' (A person with good emotional health can express all emotions appropriately, and **can maintain** a balance of emotions so that difficult emotions are not dominant.)

This is where the project comes in. Renewing and managing your emotional health is a long-term project, and one which you can maintain over time. It involves recognising unhelpful habits and gradually replacing these with healthier habits. It involves building support networks, talking about feelings, and understanding your own emotional health. It is not a one-off event, but a series of small changes which become habitual. In this way you can learn to maintain a balance of emotions.

KEY POINT: *Emotional health is both a re-building and a maintenance project.*

'Balance of Emotions'

*'BALANCE OF EMOTIONS' (A person with good emotional health can express all emotions appropriately, and can maintain a **balance of emotions** so that difficult emotions are not dominant.)*

A lot of people think that emotional health involves perpetual happiness. It doesn't. Happiness is one emotion amongst many. Emotional health involves a balance of the easier emotions like happiness and joy alongside the more difficult emotions, such as sadness and anger. Emotional health involves downs as well as ups. Recognising when your emotions have some balance is not easy. We can drift through life missing all the signs that we aren't balanced, but as you become more used to reflecting on your wellbeing it becomes habitual to look for some balance. Remember the goal is balance, not perpetual happiness.

KEY POINT: *Emotional health involves downs as well as ups.*

Putting all these ideas together brings us back to our definition. When we decide to tackle the project of our own emotional health, we are working towards balance and appropriate ways to express emotions.

> **KEY POINT:** *A person with good emotional health can express all emotions appropriately, and can maintain a balance of emotions so that difficult emotions are not dominant.*

Even difficult emotions have a purpose

Although no emotions are bad, some emotions are more difficult than others. They might be particularly painful, or frightening, or overwhelming. Some emotions might impact on your life more than others.

List two or three emotions which regularly impact your life in difficult ways:
1.
2.
3.

Did answering this question come easily to you, or did you have to dig deep?

Do any of these emotions feel out of control?

Although some emotions are difficult, they are not bad. Although these difficult emotions might seem out of control, or to be asserting a dominant influence on your life, they do have a purpose. All emotions have a purpose.

My experience is that people have often built an impression that certain feelings are 'good' and certain feelings are 'bad'. This can make dealing with them more difficult. Hiding from them, ignoring them, trying to force them out of you or trying to replace them with something else, can eventually lead to greater problems. Even difficult emotions have a job to do. A starting point for getting difficult emotions under control is to understand them, and as you begin to understand them you can let them do their job.

It's not easy understanding the intended purpose of difficult emotions, as they get caught up in the wheels of unhealthy habits, and difficult emotions often whirlpool together and muddy the waters. Sometimes we cover up one difficult emotion with a different difficult emotion. It can take a long time to unravel difficult emotions and consider where they came from and why, but it is a useful project to undertake. In VERY general terms, sadness brings comfort, anger gives us strength to solve a problem, anxiety warns us that there is something we don't feel equipped for, jealousy warns us of a threat to our social world, depression takes away motivation to allow you the comfort of not being responsible for outcomes, guilt helps us self-reflect. This is not an exact or definitive list, but it might give you a starting point. Look back on one of the difficult emotions you listed above.

What could this difficult emotion be TRYING to achieve?

This is a complex area, and there are no easy answers, but it is still a good starting point. An approach that I often take with people is to encourage them to think of their difficult emotions as warning lights, and consider what their emotions are trying to tell them.

> **KEY POINT:** *Even difficult emotions have a job to do.*

Emotions aren't naughty children

Most people fear difficult emotions. They fear being overwhelmed by them or dragged into unhappiness. What very few people do is listen to their difficult emotions. Many people go through life trying to rid themselves of all negative emotions but that is never going to happen – those emotions have a job to do and they're going to make sure that they do it. It is much more effective to learn the language of emotions and let them have their say. In this way we still have difficult emotions in our life but their hold on us is diminished. When they make us feel something, we respond to the feelings, and possibly make changes in our lives. In this way we regain some control in our lives and can work towards emotional balance.

Emotions aren't naughty children. They are very well-behaved children. They generally follow predictable patterns. They sometimes warn us about things, or protect us from things. Difficult emotions have a job to do. We need to listen to them and let them do their job. The reason these difficult emotions often grow and overwhelm us is that we try to shut them out and ignore them. And then inevitably they do become naughty children and we end up with more problems.

Lots of us find ourselves using certain emotions to cover up for other emotions. We might use anger to cover unhappiness. Or happiness to mask guilt. We might cover shame with pride. Sometimes we do this consciously, putting on a mask, and pretending everything is fine. Sometimes we do this subconsciously, acting out a certain emotion without even realising that it is actually something else we are feeling.

Management of difficult emotions is really helpful, but there will probably come a time when you want to consider what's behind them. Have we learned patterns of behaviour in our childhood? Have we absorbed traumatic events? Have we built behaviour patterns that we need to change? These big questions are best explored with a good listener. As we talk to someone else, we can begin to make sense of difficult emotions in our life.

KEY POINT: *TRY to listen to difficult emotions, rather than become frustrated with them.*

Sadness

I watched the cartoon film *Inside Out* with my children, and it blew me away. It challenged my entire approach to being a Wellbeing Lead. What I loved so much is that it highlighted something that people hadn't been talking about. In the story, the girl, Riley, thinks that she is supposed to be happy. She thinks that is what is expected of her, and so she suppresses her more difficult emotions. None of the emotions will let Sadness control Riley's emotions. The twist in the film is that when Riley's world falls apart it is only by allowing Sadness in, that she can learn to heal. It is a beautiful film and an incredibly important message.

There's a fine line to be walked between finding positivity and pretending to be happy. We can't convince our minds to be happy by pretending. Gradually building habits of authentic positivity can improve our wellbeing. Ironically, it can be through allowing ourselves the comfort of sadness that we begin to find these habits.

Sadness brings comfort. We all enjoy a sad film. And yet, somehow, many of us have convinced ourselves to hide, repress, or fear sadness. Sometimes the best thing you can do for your overall emotional wellbeing is to have a good cry. Indulge yourself in sadness, have a duvet day, and let sadness comfort you.

> **KEY POINT:** *Sadness brings comfort and can improve our wellbeing.*

Happiness

On a scale of desirable emotions happiness will always rate highly. The pursuit of happiness is many people's goal in life. There's no denying that happiness is great, but it's also important to recognise that perpetual happiness is an unrealistic goal. What is happiness anyway?

Think of five other words for happiness?
1.
2.
3.
4.
5.

These different words reflect different states of being. Emotions can be hard to define, and none more so than happiness. Pleasure and joy describe different things. Contentment is not the same as ecstasy. Of the five words you wrote down, which is the most attractive to you? If you could only have one, which one would you choose.

How responsible are you for your happiness?

Sit for a while with that question.
Don't rush into an answer.

Consider a scale.

How responsible are you for your own happiness?

100%_____0%

COMPLETELY | MOSTLY | SOMEWHAT | PARTLY | HARDLY AT ALL | NOT AT ALL

Try placing yourself on this scale.

There is no right answer. This is one of the most effective questions I've found in determining how people will approach the project of improving their emotional health.

Personally, I think it's unlikely that anyone is completely responsible for their own happiness. Circumstances have *some* impact on our happiness. But, although this extreme end of the scale seems idealistic, it still seems more helpful to recognise that our happiness isn't completely bound up with our circumstances.

> **KEY POINT:** *Happiness comes in many flavours, and all are appealing. Perpetual happiness is not the goal of wellbeing, but we could all enjoy a little more happiness in our lives.*

The Happy Man

For several years, I was known as The Happy Man because I taught happiness in schools. I went into a mainstream secondary school to teach the subject of happiness, based on my research into Positive Psychology. Sometimes people thought I was trying to teach people how to be happy, which is impossible. What I actually did in these lessons was to notice general characteristics of happy people and explore these. There are things to learn from people who have discovered patterns and habits which produce more than the average amount of happiness.

Consider these questions:

- At what age are people happiest?

- In general, are males or females happier?

- Are rich people happier?

- In society, are people becoming happier?

It's impossible to accurately measure someone's happiness, and answers are quite subjective so it is difficult to be certain about these answers. But there are huge amounts of research around the subject and some general themes emerge. We are generally at our happiest in childhood, around eight years old, and retirement, around sixty-eight. In developed countries women are generally happier, but in less developed countries, females are generally unhappier than males. Whether a country is rich or poor, average earners report the highest levels of happiness. And in Western society rates of happiness are generally falling.

Now consider your own relationship with happiness.

- How responsible do you feel for your own happiness?

- When were you at your happiest?

- What helps you find happiness?

Many people got a lot from these lessons, but there were always some who found them frustrating. Some people really bristled at the idea of thinking about happiness. I actually think that some of their objections were valid. However much I tried not to, by virtue of the fact that I was called 'The Happy Man' and involved in Positive Psychology, I inevitably conveyed an impression that happiness was the goal. This sat at odds with my wider experience of wellbeing. Happiness is not the only answer. People don't only want to be happy. I don't even think it would be good for people to be happy all the time. People aren't built to be perpetually happy. When I was known as The Happy Man, people would have a niggling suspicion that I was trying to turn them into grinning automatons. Sometimes people would resist the idea of happiness itself and then end up feeling guilty. They would then add guilt to their roster of difficult emotions. The truth is that people like being grumpy some of the time. People enjoy the self-care of sadness and the comfort of sorrow. The complicated emotions of sadness, anger, shame and irritation have important jobs to do in our lives and, as such, they shouldn't make us feel guilty. And it is worth reflecting that although these emotions can be difficult, we can 'enjoy' them as well.

> **KEY POINT:** *It can be useful to look at characteristics of happy people, but the aim isn't to be happy all the time.*

Do circumstances help?

I used to work in a place which sold lottery tickets. All day long people would be relying on the lottery for their happiness. Some weeks this little candle of hope was the only thing they were clinging on to. I always worry when people say, 'maybe I'll win the lottery'. My worry isn't what will happen if they don't win the lottery, it's what will happen if they do. I think winning the lottery must be miserable for most people. When you have convinced yourself that all your troubles are because you don't have enough money, and then money comes to you, and your problems are still there, it's quite a bleak place to be. And, to top it all, people will now be annoyed at you for being unhappy. People will have less empathy for you, and empathy is the biggest healer when it comes to our wellbeing. I think it's hard to be rich and happy. Two of the things which give us the most happiness – empathy and purpose – have been made harder for you.

I'm not sure why we all think that a change of circumstances will make us happy, because the evidence of our own eyes, and even the evidence of our own experience, tells us otherwise. We've all been in the situation where we convince ourselves that one promotion, one new thing, one dream fulfilled, or one healthy relationship will fix our problems, and it never does. And we've seen it in others too. The happiest people we know are not the ones with the best circumstances. Not at all. When we travel we see people in extraordinarily difficult circumstances, and they are often extremely happy. And we all know of the person whose circumstances seem ideal, and they're not happy. There comes a time when you just have to accept this evidence and admit to yourself that circumstances have little or no effect on happiness.

> **KEY POINT:** *Emotional health is hardly connected at all to your circumstances.*

Five things to do before breakfast

1. Stretch

2. Smile at yourself in the mirror

3. Wear something quirky, even if you take it off later

4. Stand straight, walk tall

5. Think of one thing to look forward to.

Short-term strategies

Most people have developed strategies for dealing with their wellbeing, even if they're not aware of what these are. We pick up habits of distracting ourselves or calming ourselves. Sometimes these strategies are helpful, sometimes they are unhelpful. Sometimes we know the things we do to help us deal with difficult emotions are harmful. Quite often they fall somewhere in the middle as well. We calm very difficult feelings with things which we feel ambivalent about. They probably aren't the best of things, but they are definitely better than what they are helping us deal with. I think it can be helpful to think of these as short-term strategies. Getting rid of them immediately, while we are busy with all the other aspects of thinking about our wellbeing could be too much. We have to be gentle with ourselves and focus on one thing at a time. On the other hand, it is good to name these things and recognise that they might be helpful right now as short-term strategies but eventually they will need replacing with healthier strategies.

Conversation about Wellbeing: Part One

On Sunday 20th February a group of men sat down to discuss their wellbeing. Ages ranged from nineteen to forty-four. We were all from different backgrounds, and we didn't all know each other, although some of us were already friends. The one thing we all had in common was that we were all regulars at different nights in Idle Games Club in Paignton, either as board gamers or role players. I have anonymised the conversations but, so that you can follow who said what, I have attributed different superhero names to all the participants. We were: Batman, Ant Man, Aquaman, Superman, Spider-man, Captain America and Iron Man. Chairing the meeting was Dr X. Suffice to say that, for a group of board gamers and role players, the conversation about who was which superhero took nearly as long as the conversation around wellbeing, but I've skipped that here. There was also pizza. In this first part of the conversation Iron Man talks about his dislike of sharing his feelings, and Batman talks about things he does to help with difficult memories, although he knows these things are not necessarily healthy in the long run. There's also a mention of Imposter Syndrome which comes up a few times in the conversation.

I started by asking the question, 'How often do you think about your own wellbeing?'

Batman started us off.

Batman: *Not as often as I should.*

Ant Man: *I'd agree with that wholeheartedly.*

Batman: *I've got people I need to take care of, the wife and the kids, so their wellbeing comes before mine.*

Ant Man: *Same here, I've got people to take care of, and a girlfriend with, in her own words, poor mental health as well.*

Iron Man: *Likewise, my little girl, and my wife, suffer with anxiety quite badly, so...*

Batman: *You suffer quite badly.*

Iron Man: *Well, not as much.*

Batman: *No, but recently I've been the one you've fallen back on.*

Iron Man: *Yeah, recently I have fallen back on you...*

Batman: *But that's fine, we all need people to fall back on.*

Dr. X: *We're supposed to, right.*

Batman: *Yeah.*

Iron Man: *And it's not like I do it often, and it's only...*

Batman: *I know, it's only about one particular thing.*

Iron Man: *I'm not one for telling people stuff. I am one of those Neanderthal men that don't like talking about stuff.*

Batman: *I think most people don't like talking about it in a public forum.*

(Spider-man, Aquaman, and Ant Man all agree.)

Iron Man: *I don't like, I don't know, even if it's one-on-one. I'm very like, 'I'll be fine.'*

Batman: *That's why I was hoping that Hulk would come because Hulk is one of those people that straight up will not... he is just one of those people that does not talk about it. Like, at all. And I was looking forward to being like, so Hulk... And poking him to get him to talk about stuff. But I knew he wouldn't! I knew deep down.*

Dr. X: *Do you talk about it less with people when they themselves don't talk about it? And if people do talk about it, do you feel freer to talk about it yourself?*

(Aquaman, Iron Man and Spiderman all say no.)

Iron Man: *I don't like measuring up. I don't want to be, 'we've just talked about you, so now let's talk about me.'*

Batman: *I mean in a way that's the thing with conversational skills.*

Iron Man: *That's how it works, I get it.*

Batman: *But that doesn't necessarily mean that if someone has talked about their own problems, you have to talk about yours. Sometimes you can just divert the subject completely, which some people do. That's fine. As long as you've got someone to talk to about different subjects, just to help you.*

Iron Man: *Do you talk to your wife much?*

Batman: *Yes, I talk to my wife a lot. She's my best friend, literally. That's the person I go to for any number of things. Including emotional stuff. I've suffered from depression. I've suffered from anxiety. I still do to a certain extent. I suffer from what you'd call Imposter Syndrome, where I don't feel I deserve the praise I get for things that I do. Over the years I've learned to cope. I've got coping mechanisms. But then there are also trauma issues that I have where I end up overeating as a trigger for anything I've suffered from, whether it be bullying or any number of different things which cause me to go into what might become a spiral into depression. It's better for me to overeat and not go into that depression that I know would cause me a lot more harm. The other option is to eat, which is obviously causing me physical harm. Let's be fair, I'm overweight and that's not a good thing.*

In this conversation, Batman recognises that overeating is a strategy to deal with all manner of things which impact his wellbeing. He recognises that it is not the healthiest strategy in the long term, but he also recognises that stopping now would leave him somewhat defenceless to deal with many other things. There are many unhealthy habits we develop to shelter us from the pain of more difficult things. Comfort eating, drinking too much, marital affairs, drugs and reckless behaviour would be some common examples, but there are more.

> *What unhealthy strategies have you built up to mask or comfort difficult feelings?*

In this conversation, Batman recognises that comfort eating won't be good for his wellbeing in the long run, but the project of improving our wellbeing is a long-term one, and sometimes we need to pick our battles. At present, simply naming and being aware of this issue is a good start. As people's overall wellbeing improves, we can gain more energy to deal with these short-term strategies. Short-term strategies can be all kinds of things. What they have in common is that we know they're not healthy in the long run. We know that if we let them carry on then they themselves become the problem.

> **KEY POINT:** *Most of us end up with coping strategies which probably aren't helpful in the long-term, but naming them and being aware of them is a good start.*

Warning lights

I find that a helpful way to understand and deal with difficult emotions is to consider them as warning lights.

Imagine you're driving alone along a quiet road at night. You didn't bring your phone. All of a sudden you see a warning light on your car. It's not one you recognise, and you haven't got the manual to check.

Be honest, what would you do?

A. Get angry

B. Anxiously try to ignore it

C. Panic and stop immediately

D. Pull over in a safe place and try to fix it

E. Pull over in a safe place and try to find a way to get help.

Difficult emotions are like the warning lights on your car. They don't feel good, but they have a job to do. Some responses are more helpful than others.

A. Getting angry is hardly ever going to help in these circumstances. (There are times in life when anger is really helpful. It can give us adrenaline to quickly solve issues of unfairness, but that doesn't apply here.) The anger will only make us less able to cope with the situation. If we are already struggling with difficult emotions, anger can add more problems.

B. I fear that this is the choice that I would most likely take, but it's not a great choice. (There are times in life when anxiety is helpful. It can focus our thoughts and make us aware of things which we may have overlooked. But in the situation above, it wouldn't help at all.) We'd be focusing all our attention on a problem we're already aware of, without doing anything to solve it. This happens a lot in life. People try to get rid of anxiety, or distract themselves from it, rather than considering what the anxiety is alerting them to.

C. In many ways, this is a better choice in the car. At least you would have stopped, and the problems won't get worse. The difficulty here is that panic can be quite debilitating. It can make it difficult to know what to do next. It's really common for people to panic at the first sign of emotional overload. People fear difficult emotions, rather than listening to them, and this fear can make them unable to deal with what life is throwing at them.

D. Well done for pulling over. Good. You may or may not be able to fix it, but it's worth having a look. At the first signs of difficult emotions, just pull over. Find a space for peace and quiet, and wait till you're feeling a bit calmer before having a think about why you're feeling that way. You may not know, but it's not done any harm to have a think, and at least you pulled over to a safe place.

E. Very good. I admire your choice. Of course, this is the best option in the car. If you don't recognise the warning light, you're probably not going to be able to fix things yourself so you will seek out help at the first opportunity. Think of your emotional world like this. At the first signs of difficult emotions, pull over and seek help. As soon as you are able to, find a place or activity which calms you, and wait till you feel calmer. Then find someone to talk to. A friend, a family member, or even a stranger. Talking helps.

In this car analogy, the first good decision is to pull over to a safe place. As you don't recognise the warning light, it would be foolish to keep going. You don't have a phone or manual to work out what is going on. If you have a good understanding of engines, you might be able to work out what is going on by lifting the bonnet. But, if not, then you will need some help and support. Sometimes, just by having someone to discuss the issue with we find it easier to make sense of it.

Conversation about Wellbeing: Part Two

Our real-life superheroes continue discussing their wellbeing. In this part we talk about opening up about feelings and why some people find this difficult.

Dr. X: *Everyone who has spoken so far has said that they don't particularly check in with their own wellbeing. Is there anyone here who does?*

Captain America: *Yes.*

Dr. X: *How do you do that?*

Captain America: *I think it's quite easy, because I'm single.*

All: *Don't we know it!*

Captain America: *I think it's just a thing I've developed over time. I've always been a person to reminisce and ruminate.*

Superman: *Overthink?*

Captain America: *Definitely, 100 per cent. I look back over emotions and conversations. Of recent, I've been talking to people about it. But, previously I was by myself figuring it out because with men it's not really a discussion, it's not something that I've wanted to open up about. But I think it's also the maturity of people at those moments. And that's probably the most difficult thing, when you might have early trauma in your life and it's difficult to communicate with people, especially in the teenage years.*

Dr. X: *And yet all the advice says, do talk about those things. I don't want to stereotype, but, as a general rule, women I know do talk about these things.*

General murmurs of agreement from Batman, Aquaman, Spiderman, Superman and Iron Man.

Iron Man: *It's not taboo anymore.*

Ant Man: *I'll disagree.*

Captain America: *Also disagree because I know a certain someone, female, who had an incident they didn't talk about for half a year, to anyone, and there's someone else who doesn't talk about their feelings.*

Dr X: *I definitely agree it's not all. You disagreed too Ant Man.*

Ant Man: *Much the same as Captain America said. My girlfriend, the love if my life, has had trauma, including traumatic birth, and her body doesn't feel like hers anymore, but she clamps down her feelings. It's only after therapy she's started. I also started therapy, which I'll say I've finished after two years, although I'm not sure you ever finish, you just pause it for a while then go back to it. Only after that we were able to talk to each other properly about that sort of stuff, and if it wasn't for another close mate of mine that I've just unloaded my life onto I wouldn't have anyone to talk to, but therapy has basically taught me that instead of saying 'I'm fine,' I can say 'I'm not fine.' That was the most useful thing that came out of that. My girlfriend is still pretty quiet about things, but she had a pretty traumatic childhood. Lots of things have happened to her since, and she doesn't know who she is anymore. If it wasn't for her therapist, and lately me, saying there's no judgement here, I'm not going anywhere. Just talk to me.*

Superman: *I think that's really important. We call it toe-time in our house.*

Iron Man: *Why toe-time?*

Superman: *The first time it happened we sat on the landing, feet out, touching. And we had a very frank conversation, and it was exactly that, 'I'm not going anywhere, just talk.' You need a level of trust in whoever you talk to. You can have toe-time with anyone, but you need that level of trust in that person. We also have mobile toe-time when we go for a long walk and do it. I think it's very, very important for checking in with your wellbeing. Sometimes for me that takes place as part of that conversation. I check in with myself as part of the conversation. I think about how am I actually feeling?*

Dr. X: *I have written this book for anyone that has ever struggled to open up about their feelings, whether male or female. I do think that some of us, when we are struggling, don't know how to begin. What do we do when the person asks us if we're fine and we're not fine? How does that go?*

Captain America: *Different people might have different behaviours. When I'm in a relationship I have other things to focus on and then I don't focus on myself as much. Like Batman, Ant Man and Iron Man have said. But when I'm out of the relationship I realise – oh right, there was a lot going on. But some people can do that as part of the relationships. Like toe-time, which Superman has realised he can do as part of the relationship.*

Iron Man: *I know my wife is going through stuff, so I don't want to add any more. If I'm feeling crappy, I'm just feeling crappy, I'll get over it. Because I know that she's... not. With some people I know, it's not just a case of getting over it, so I won't put anything upon them. I'm very, very on the side of 'everyone is going through something' and I agree with that, but this is my thing.*

Batman: *You seem to be weighing stuff up as levels. Weighing one thing against the other.*

Iron Man: *That's how I see it. And I know I'm a very angry person. I get quite angry very quickly, so if I haven't had a day to myself, which hardly ever happens, I'll just lash out.*

Dr. X: *But, knowing that about yourself, is kind of checking in with yourself. If you know that those times are getting close, and you know those things will happen unless you take time for yourself, then that is checking in with yourself.*

Iron Man: *But I don't call it that.*

Captain America: *It's just hard in the moment because you don't realise until you lash out.*

Dr. X: *That's the key. If you can become a little bit more aware of those things before they happen.*

Captain America: *So it's like realising you can see the water boiling before it spills over.*

In this conversation the analogy is noticing water boiling before it spills over, which is a fantastic analogy. It's the same idea, of seeing the difficult feelings as warning lights and heeding the warning. This approach is absolutely key to coping with difficult emotions. The world can be confusing and overwhelming. It can be stressful and tiring. It can be upsetting and infuriating. Sometimes it is all these things at once. When difficult emotions come, we don't always know what is going on and why. We are not at our best to cope with things. We have a huge warning light flashing in our mind, telling us to STOP! Just stop! In this conversation the men either crashed or stopped. When they stopped, they opened up in various ways to various people. We had Captain America regularly self-reflecting. Ant-Man opening up to a close mate. Superman having toe-time with his partner. Then we have Iron Man who doesn't think he does stop and check-in with himself and maybe does need to build more opportunities into his life to stop and self-reflect, or open up to others. It can be hard to build these habits into life. It can feel easier to keep crashing through life with the habits we've developed, but in the end that is not a great long-term strategy. As soon as it's safe, or possible, just stop. Find a place, or activity which calms you and let it calm you. Then, talk to someone.

As you become used to seeing difficult emotions as alarm bells, or recognising when the water is close to boiling, the healthier responses we develop of taking time to stop, of doing calming activities, of opening up to others or self-reflecting on what is going on and why, become healthier habits for us.

> **KEY POINT:** *Think of difficult emotions as warning lights, telling you to get to a safe place and get help.*

Panic!

Difficult emotions are warning lights. And, responding to warnings, some of us panic. For a lot of us our first response to difficult feelings is one of panic. Some people have a natural leaning towards panic.

> *When was the last time you panicked about anything?*
>
> *What did it feel like?*

Panic in emotional health is often the body's first response; it might look like worry, or anxiety, or stress, or fear. Or with other people it might look like anger, or compulsive behaviour, or depression, or guilt. Panic in emotions is when any emotion overwhelms us, dominates us, and makes us act out-of-character. This is panic.

> *In your emotional life, what feelings regularly overwhelm you?*
>
> *In your emotional life, what feelings cause you to act out-of-character? (this may be the same answer).*

Panic overwhelms us; it washes over our body and we feel it everywhere. It takes us over, and makes it difficult to think rationally. Just when we need our best response we respond in a panic, and this is rarely helpful. The trouble with panic is that it makes it harder to act rationally. When we recognise things as panic, we have more chance of dealing with them. There is usually no point in dealing with the situation causing the panic until you have dealt with the panic itself. If we are going to do anything about the situation which is causing the panic, we need to be on our 'A' game, which we won't be while we are panicking. When you feel panic rising in you, recognise it as an alarm bell, and stop. Recognise it as an alarm, not a rational response. Do something calming, open up to someone, or self-reflect on what is happening. Don't try and tackle the situation causing the panic, until you deal with the panic itself.

KEY POINT: *Your natural instinct might be to panic, but seek out calm when you feel the rise of difficult feelings.*

How to be a brain surgeon

Emotions exist. They are not some vague ephemeral things. People can talk about difficult feelings as if they are 'all in the mind'. They are also in the brain and the body. They are actual neuro-logical brain states. In your brain neurons may fire up; in your body various things may happen to your muscles, skin and organs. Let's consider one part of your brain called the amygdala. It's a small almond shaped part of your brain, which is sometimes known as the reptilian brain.

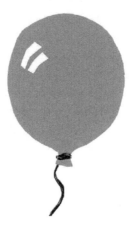

Imagine that this balloon represents your brain. This balloon is nice and plump and full of air. Your brain is running at full strength and your emotions are helping you make sense of the world. All is well. In my analogy, the amygdala is the mouth of the balloon. The amygdala manages your fight, flight, freeze response. There may be times in your life when this fight, flight, freeze response is needed. It short-circuits your thinking brain and helps you to react instinctively, rather than through logical thought. This may prove very useful. Imagine someone holding the balloon by its mouth and then letting it go. The balloon whizzes away. This is you instinctively reacting with fight, flight or freeze. Your higher thinking brain is not involved in this decision.

Various things can make our amygdala wired for fight, flight, freeze. These can include a long-term build-up of unacknowledged emotions, trauma, difficult emotions which have not been talked through, and a long time dealing with emotions in unhealthy ways. These patterns and habits mean that the amygdala builds a habit of being ready to be triggered.

Imagine me pinching the end of the balloon while it screeches. That represents your amygdala screaming an alarm to the rest of your brain. When your amygdala has built a habit of holding, denying, or ignoring difficult emotions, it causes emotions to bypass your logical thinking brain, and you are unable to consider things carefully. Instead things go straight to panic mode. This is like the air escaping the balloon. You end up like a reptile, not able to consider whether threats are real, but instinctively being wired for fight, flight or freeze.

Our balloon hasn't burst. It is simply deflated, and can be re-inflated. This is like your brain. It can be healed. You can become a brain surgeon, and heal your overwhelmed brain. When we feel tense, or anxious, or stressed or angry, or miserable or guilty, or other un-checked difficult emotions, they can build and build to the point where logical, considered thought becomes impossible. The warning light has been flashing for a while and we've been ignoring it. The warning light is telling us to pull over in a safe place and ask for help. The safe place will calm us for a while, but we need to express our feelings in order to re-inflate the balloon.

> **KEY POINT:** *When the amygdala feels overwhelmed it will cause your feelings to by-pass the thinking brain.*

Your sixth sense

How do you know when you're hungry? Eventually your tummy might rumble but, before that, how do you know? Or thirsty, how quickly do you know? Or tired, what do you notice first? Most of us are reasonably good at eventually recognising these signals. We could become better at it.

Our bodies have a sixth sense: the sense of interoception, our own sense of recognising and regulating our body's signals. Hunger, thirst, tiredness, temperature. Here's where it becomes even more relevant. Our interoceptors can also recognise and regulate our emotional health, if only we learned to listen to them more.

Our sixth sense of interoception listens to signals in our body. Some of these are reasonably obvious, like hunger, but some are more elusive, such as emotional health, stress levels and life balance. We're not all tuned in to these signals at the same level. How tuned in you are to your emotional wellbeing? Interoceptors will have an effect on your wellbeing.

The good news is that we can become more attuned to these things. Listening carefully to our own signals becomes easier the more we do it. When you start to think of your difficult emotions as warning lights you become more attuned to your interoceptors. By listening to difficult emotions, taking notice of them and finding ways to restore wellbeing, we are getting used to using our interoceptors. Gradually, listening to them becomes easier and we automatically start building healthy habits and rhythms. We recognise the warning lights of difficult emotions quickly, we slow down, rest, and reflect and use our new habits of self-care to restore our wellbeing.

Before we reach this point we are often extraordinarily deaf to our interoceptors. I've done it myself. I had NO idea that when my anxiety levels were on the rise, I would hum the theme song to Last of The Summer Wine, until someone pointed it out. No idea at all! Now it's one of my alarms. It's important to consider these things and take time to self-reflect.

> *What are some of the signals that you are becoming overwhelmed?*
>
> *How quickly do you respond to these signals?*
>
> *Where do you first notice difficult emotions in your body?*

You may not be able to answer these questions. Listening to our interoceptors takes practice. It doesn't come easily. Sometimes you will need to work backwards from the point when you have already become overwhelmed. Respond by stopping, finding calming activities and thinking about your feelings, but, specifically, try to chart the things you felt in your mind and body just before you became overwhelmed.

Being well rested will help with your sensitivity to your interoceptors. A lot of us need to listen more carefully to our interoceptors to gain a more attuned sixth sense on when we can make small changes to increase our overall wellbeing.

KEY POINT: *A key to managing your emotional health is becoming more attuned to your interoceptors.*

Love Yourself

If you spend some time looking for emotional health advice online, it won't be long before you come across someone telling you to 'love yourself'. It's important to love yourself. I agree. But, what if you can't! What if you don't know how. This is where the advice seems to fall down. I've never seen any advice on HOW. I want to address this, with a reasonably simple principle which can make all the difference. That principle is this:

We love what we care for

This simple truth is incredibly important. It goes to the heart of what love is, but it also gives us a way in to learning to love ourselves.

First, a story.

When I was younger my nan gave me a scruffy rat as a Christmas present. I was not keen on rats. I'd been bitten by one once and I'd learned to be nervous around them. I was not a fan. I did not like this rat. I could have left things at that and half-heartedly looked after the rat till it died unloved in a cage. But I loved my nan, and that seemed disrespectful to her. I decided that even if I didn't love the rat I could care for it well. I lavished care on my rat. Good food, attention and clean bedding. And I learned to love it.

If I had half-heartedly looked after it, I would never have developed love for it, but we love what we care for. The very act of caring creates love and that's how humans are built.

What things, people or pets do you regularly take care of?

This principle applies to self-care, which can eventually turn into self-love. We can't manufacture self-love. But we CAN manufacture self-care. Self-care is an act of the will, not an emotional state. Consider all the effort you put into caring for others. You care because you love them, but you also love them because you care. This relationship works both ways. Even if you don't FEEL love for yourself, if you act as if you do, then by caring you will walk towards loving yourself more.

> **KEY POINT:** *If you have low self-esteem, or you just don't know how to love yourself, one way to change this is to practise self-care.*

Why talking about feelings helps

It can be quite a common response to think that sharing our feelings only makes them worse. Or we can be too embarrassed to share our feelings. Or we think that we can cope on our own. Or we have learnt ways to ignore them or distract ourselves from difficult feelings. Or we think that sharing feelings isn't very 'manly'. But talking about feelings does help.

Conversation about Wellbeing: Part Three

Our real-life superheroes continue discussing their wellbeing. Here we touch on listening to others and empathy.

Aquaman: *I feel like men and women's mental health is near identical, and the reason that men's mental health often reaches that boiling point is societal norms of how it's viewed. In my life I've always been told 'man up'. Get on with it. You don't have time to be wasting. You need to do this. And that can also be said to me if I'm doing stuff to help with my mental health.*

Dr. X: *It's a shame because you're so much younger than me, and I hoped things were changing. Do we still think the stereotype still exists?*

General murmurs of agreement.

Batman: *That isn't going anywhere soon.*

Aquaman: *I also think it's how generations teach other generations.*

Batman: *I think, on a generational level, some generations think they've had it harder than others. But if you look at the facts, every generation has those moments.*

Iron Man: *I've got my dad's anger.*

Batman: *And I know I've picked up on things, from what I've been told.*

Superman: *Normal is what's normal in your life. If you are beaten for a long time, that becomes normal for you. Who's to say you should know any different?*

Captain America: *But it's noticing it.*

Superman: *Unless you turn a corner and say that wasn't right.*

Captain America: *You might look at another family and realise.*

Iron Man: *How do you measure up? If you tell me about this stuff, that could be such a serious thing. I'm not comparing, but that could be a serious thing, but I might not know it's a serious thing. It might not look it to me.*

Captain America: *It comes down to how empathetic you are. Maybe, if someone tells you something, you don't see it as anything.*

Iron Man: *There was a time when I might have just called you names. And I have learnt to reel it in a bit. But before I would have just said, 'it's just names mate, you're taking it the wrong way'. I wouldn't have known then that it wasn't. Sorry, I'm not belittling anything you've been through.*

Dr. X: *Earlier you said you wouldn't want to open up to someone because it would be a burden, but I want you to think back to when someone has opened up to you. If someone has opened up to you, were you pleased?*

Most people murmur agreement.

Ant Man: *Personally, yes.*

Iron Man: *It depends how long they've known you.*

Ant Man: *If it was a random stranger I'd be concerned.*

Dr. X: *If it was a mate...*

Ant Man: *Then yes. Twice in my life I've been at horrific low points and my friends were there for me. I would have gone off the rails, swum in the sea or something. They were there for me, and I'd hope I could be there for someone else.*

Captain America: *I wouldn't even mind a stranger.*

Iron Man: *You're a caring person...*

Captain America: *It's having that knowledge that everyone is struggling. I asked someone at work, and it turned out they were going through big struggles and* *by listening to them we became close friends. I have no problems even if it was stranger.*

Batman: *Take the scenario where you go out for a drink with work mates. You don't know them too well, they're acquaintances. And then a few drinks in and someone gets upset. I would happily go up to them and say, 'what's the matter?' I've had it happen to me, and I've done it to other people. It's sort of like an empathy puddle. Not the deepest of things but shallow enough you can splash about. And it is this thing where you can still show some level of empathy and just listen and that's often enough for people.*

Aquaman: *I would be glad, mostly, that they'd have enough trust to open up to me. Then I'd know I could trust them with my feelings at a later time.*

Spiderman: *I've had many friends open up to me. A friend of mine with anxiety and depression opens up to me. I do allow them just to let it out.*

Superman: *I think I'd be alright, but it is also a burden. I'd think, 'am I the only person they've spoken to about this?' Because if I'm not, fair enough, they're looking to vent. But if I am, there's the panic of what on earth do I do with this information. There's an emerging way forward, which is validating someone's feelings. And this is a very British thing which we do not do. We always go, 'but it's not as bad as this'. 'At least it's not...'*

Aquaman: *That's a common problem.*

Superman: *What we need to do is flip that on its head and say, 'that sucks!' 'What a shame, that's terrible for you.' If you validate that person's feelings, they don't feel put down.*

Most of us understand that talking helps. And we might even understand that empathy helps. But few people understand why.

It is through sharing feelings that the amygdala will start to heal the brain. It is by talking, and sharing our feelings, that we can re-inflate the balloon of our brains. We tend to know this instinctively, but then talk ourselves out of it. Take the above conversation. All of these people have been the talker and the listener, and they all know it does help, but sometimes they talk themselves out of this. Maybe it all seems too simple. It's a simple principle but a complicated process. Most of the people in this conversation have highlighted times when being able to open up to someone has stopped them going off the rails.

Why does talking about feelings help?

The first reason is quite simple. When we express our feelings as words, through talking or writing, we have to use our higher-thinking brains. The reptilian brain doesn't have higher skills like language. Expressing our deep feelings in ways that others can understand adds a layer of complexity which our instinctive amygdala can never reach. This automatically moves some of the feelings from the fight, fight, freeze response into the more logical higher thinking brain.

The second reason why sharing our feelings is so important is more complicated, but it is incredibly important. The single most effective thing at healing your brain, when it has become deflated like the balloon, is empathy. The thing your overwhelmed brain needs more than any other is for someone to listen and understand. Nothing is more effective than this. Empathy can change your entire brain state. When someone listens and understands it makes you feel lighter. It changes your thought patterns. You can approach life differently.

*When did someone last listen to
you empathetically?*

*Who is the most empathetic person
you know?*

*When did you last have the chance to
listen empathetically to someone?*

How easy or difficult did you find it?

People describe empathy as walking in someone else's shoes, but I find this image unhelpful. No-one needs to share your experiences. They just need to listen and understand. That will heal you. My favourite description of the empathetic listening response is sitting comfortably with someone else's emotions.

When someone sits comfortably with your overwhelming emotions it calms you, it normalises your experiences, and it quietens your amygdala to make it easier to access your logical brain. If someone will sit comfortably while you express your deep feelings, then you will have met the greatest brain surgeon in the world. The brain heals itself.

And the beauty is that you can do the same. When we empathise with someone, we can calm the reptilian part of their brain and heal the higher brain. In this way, you too, can be the greatest brain surgeon in the world.

> **KEY POINT:** *One of the best ways to find emotional help is through talking to someone who listens and understands.*

Why advice might be the last thing you need

Part of the reason why people are reluctant to seek help is that they misunderstand the healing process. People think that when people are struggling, they need advice. And yet, when people are struggling with difficult emotions, advice might not help. People sometimes avoid sharing their feelings because they don't trust other people's advice. Tragically, lots of people also feel uncomfortable listening to other people talking about difficult feelings because they feel unqualified to offer advice. This sense is often right. Advice can sometimes undermine empathy.

Five tips for instant self-care

1. Call your best friend and talk about your feelings

2. Eat some fruit

3. Have a long bath

4. Accept things you can't change

5. Deep abdominal breathing.

Consider this. My eleven year old daughter comes to me with some friendship struggles at school. My first instinct is to offer advice. It doesn't matter if my advice is good or bad. Because I have offered advice, she storms out of the room shouting 'you just don't understand.' And she's right. I haven't offered her my understanding. By offering advice, I've shrunk her complicated emotional world into a small box of my own partial understanding. Much better would be for me to simply listen and understand.

> **KEY POINT:** *Advice can sometimes work against emotional healing.*

Is recovery possible?

Nine times out of ten, when I help someone with their emotional health, they have an unvoiced hope that someone will unearth a hidden source of their troubles. They might have seen fictionalised examples of treatment where the helper uncovers some hidden trauma, and this discovery brings breakthrough. Be honest with yourself, have you ever wished that someone could unearth one source of all your wellbeing troubles? In my experience, this almost never happens. Recovery rarely looks like this. Recovery of emotional health is a slow and frustrating project, not a quick fix.

I understand the instinct to find one source of all wellbeing struggles. I have done the same with my physical health. I remember when I was growing thinner and thinner, and my heart was racing so hard it kept me awake at night, and I was growing weaker and weaker. When I was diagnosed with an over-active thyroid I was initially really pleased to have a name to everything. I was amazed that one thing was the source of all my health troubles and it could be dealt with. But then things got complicated! The medication to calm my thyroid made me sluggish. I thought I had a natural energy but then it seemed that some of this was actually due to a health condition. I also realised that I would have to take medication for life, and this was not easy for me.

With emotional health it's even more problematic. Our mental health struggles can be even more closely connected with our identity than our physical struggles. There was no easy answer to how much of me was due to my over-active thyroid. Some things were coping strategies, some things were the result of hormonal imbalance. I have worked along-side doctors to get my hormones balanced and my thyroid under control, and I'm incredibly grateful for their expertise. Recovery of wellbeing IS possible. It absolutely is. But it's never simple. Many people have this desire to find one quick fix, or to have things labelled so they can be understood. This desire to diagnose wellbeing struggles, to label them, and then understand them can actually get in the way of recovery. Most emotional health struggles are the result of years of unhealthy habits and coping strategies. There might be hidden trauma but, even if there is, it will have become part of the furniture of your brain. The habits you build up over time become well-worn paths in your brain. Even as you notice these and start to take different paths, your habits will keep re-surfacing. Habits take a long time to break. But they CAN be broken.

Five lifestyle changes to make

1. Prioritise sleep

2. Prioritise healthy eating

3. Actively try to listen to others more

4. Spend more time outside every day

5. Find a new recovery pastime.

This is one of the most difficult aspects of emotional health recovery. Just when you are feeling at your weakest, you have to face the prospect of a slow and frustrating up-hill struggle.

Recovery involves an acceptance that healing will actually come in a series of mundane actions repeated over and over again. One of the reasons that emotional health is so hard to face is because the recovery involves daily grind and motivation, but many forms of emotional health lower people's basic motivation.

This all sounds bleak but there is a good side. The positive side of this is that the small things actually do help. The positive side is that some recovery is possible. Each prosaic step brings barely noticed recoveries each time.

> **KEY POINT:** *Recovery is slow and difficult, but it is possible.*

PART THREE
STARTING THE PROJECT

It's a habit!

The starting point of this project to improve wellbeing and emotional health is to replace unhealthy coping strategies with healthier coping strategies.

We all have habits. A habit is an acquired behaviour or thought pattern that someone has repeated so many times that it has become subconscious. We create habits to make life easier. We tie our shoes a certain way. We have a morning routine that is the same almost every day. Most people even brush their teeth a particular way. We engage in habits without thinking, which frees our brains up to focus on other things. We programme our life and put it on autopilot so that we aren't so overwhelmed by every little decision and task, but sometimes we programme reactions without thinking. Some habits are positive and promote healthy patterns of happiness and growth. We also pick up negative habits that are destructive and undermine our happiness and emotional health. Improving our wellbeing involves replacing bad habits with good ones.

The lifestyle changes in Project Emotional Health are both simple and complicated. They look simple because they are easy to explain. But they are also complicated because they involve lifestyle changes and consistency. These things only start to work when they become ingrained habits.

Five large projects to try

1. Sign up for an allotment

2. Couch to 5k running

3. Tidy and organise the house

4. Adopt a pet

5. Start volunteering regularly.

A lot of my job involves helping people to understand emotional first aid. And it's the simple things which help. I wish there were magic wands but there rarely are. The things which help are the daily things. One thing which helps is to start talking about feelings more, and changing the habit of keeping things inside. It is the daily motivational cost of avoiding the unhealthy habits and the further motivational cost of replacing them with healthy strategies. And all the time recognising that your motivation is probably at an all-time low. Each step is helping. Your mental health struggles probably established themselves slowly, so they can be dismantled slowly. But they can be dismantled. Recovery is possible.

> **KEY POINT:** *Recovery involves replacing unhealthy thought habits with healthy thought habits.*

The first step is the hardest

A phrase which I have been using to describe recovery of emotional health is 'project'. This word acknowledges the day-to-day nature of recovery. It recognises each step on the journey as being important. Each and every step towards your goal is part of the recovery.

The first step is the one which orientates the recovery. The first step is the one which costs the most. The first step is the one where a direction is chosen. From the moment of the first step the recovery project has begun. Even if you slip back, even if you slip back further than you started, if you have orientated yourself towards recovery then the project is already happening.

I am so proud of you for starting this project. Learning to manage your emotional health and wellbeing is an orientation towards a goal of self-improvement.

> **KEY POINT:** *From the moment of the first step the recovery project has begun.*

Sorry for being annoying

Each person, whether they acknowledge it or not, has certain areas of emotional health which hold them back. No one has life completely sorted. We are all on a journey. In an ideal world, people would embrace their own mental health blueprint. They would proudly own their characteristics as something which makes them special and unique. In addition to this, they would begin to recognise the ways in which their own watermark brings joys as well as struggles into their world. It's so hard to do that. It's particularly hard to do that when mental ill-health often undermines self-esteem.

Or when it attacks motivation. Or when the recovery and management involve so much day-to-day grind. Or when the struggles make so much daily life seem like a mountain to climb. It can be hard to smell the roses when you're piling on the manure. This can make some of the advice seem really annoying. I know! I've been there too, and all I can do is apologise. It's annoying when someone tells you to open up about your feelings. That's why I've tried to explain why this is necessary. It's annoying when people remind you to look after yourself. Just because this advice is annoying, it doesn't make it wrong. Recovery needs certain activators. Things like hope, motivation and purpose are needed to trigger recovery. The language of hope, motivation and purpose can seem trite, but that doesn't make it wrong. Sometimes you need to keep reminding yourself about these things because hope, motivation and purpose are the very things which much mental illness attacks. Wellbeing involves finding small examples of hope, and using these things to activate the daily grind of managing your emotional health, and then regularly reminding yourself that the things you are doing help, even when they seem annoying. It's hard, and you might need people around who recognise and acknowledge why it is so hard. And that it's alright to recognise and acknowledge that it is hard, which it is. It's alright to acknowledge these things, but then it's also helpful to remind yourself that they ARE helping. It is this that you need to keep coming back to. It is hard because it is possible.

> **KEY POINT:** *Recovery is hard, but possible.*

The catch-22

The phrase catch-22 describes a situation which traps you in a circle of contradiction. I can't do A because of B, but I can't do B because of A. An example would include a job-seeker who could only find jobs which needed experience but couldn't get the experience because no-one would give them a job.

One of the draining aspects of low emotional health is that it can trap you in a catch-22 situation. Low emotional health can cause individuals to lack motivation, hope and energy. But these are the very things the individual needs most to keep them going through the tough times. Project Recovery needs to be fuelled by motivation, hope and energy, but the person who needs Project Recovery often lacks these very things. This can cause immense frustration. It's downright annoying. But don't despair because recognising and understanding the catch-22 can arm you against it. The frustration and tension of the catch-22 can be undermined by acknowledging it. It is the catch-22 which can make it annoying when people try to help. Their ideas and advice can seem both annoyingly simple and frustratingly difficult at the same time. The logical part of your brain may recognise that there are annoyingly 'simple' things you could do to help your emotional health, but the emotional part of your brain will make these things seem either incredibly difficult or completely pointless.

Low emotional health can attack the areas of the brain which support motivation, energy and hope. The things which are needed to help recovery become difficult to do.

Understanding this catch-22 can help. It can help people to see that small steps will help, even if these things seem annoyingly simple in themselves. Some relatively simple ideas can help, but that doesn't make them simple to do. They still take effort and motivation, which are in short supply.

There are lots of things which can help people to recover good emotional health; it's not just the 'simple' things, but it is the 'simple' things which get undermined by the catch-22.

These 'simple' things can include:

Eating well, exercising, walking, talking to people, helping people, being encouraging, getting out of bed, being in nature, getting a good night's sleep, resting.

- When your brain convinces itself that these things won't help, that's the catch-22 talking.

- When these ideas seem annoying, that's the catch-22 talking.

- When you convince yourself that you don't need these things, that's the catch-22 talking.

- When these things start to seem impossible, that's the catch-22 talking.

Low emotional health makes these things difficult, but not impossible.

> **KEY POINT:** *Recognising the catch-22 can arm you against it.*

Recovery pastimes

Everyone that I know who has focused on their own wellbeing and prioritised their own emotional health has found one or two activities which help more than anything else. These activities might calm them, or focus them, or make them feel content. I call these activities 'recovery pastimes'. Finding and developing recovery pastimes is crucial to recovery and management of wellbeing. Our superheroes talk about things which have helped them to find balance in their wellbeing.

Conversation about Wellbeing: Part Four

Our real-life superheroes continue to talk about their wellbeing. I have asked them here to say one thing which helps with their wellbeing. Bear in mind that this is a group of people who have come together through a shared love of board games and role-playing games. Not surprisingly these activities feature highly.

Dr X: *What helps most with your wellbeing?*

Ant Man: *Coming here on Wednesdays. For mental health generally in lockdown I really struggled to get out of the house. So, playing Dungeons and Dragons. I also miss taking photos, I've got an epic digital camera. It takes wonderful photos. So that's my mental health goal. To sling it over my shoulder and just get out and about.*

Captain America: *I don't know.*

Iron Man: *You speak to someone though, does that help?*

Captain America: *It's difficult at the same time.*

Ant Man: *It's like a 50-50, even when speaking with people.*

Superman: *I've heard that therapy can be absolutely... you can come away feeling terrible.*

Bat Man: *You need the right person though.*

Iron Man: *You may need to go through it to get out of it.*

Bat Man: *I've heard from so many people that it took them so long to find the right person.*

Superman: *That's awful.*

Captain America: *When you look at your wellbeing it's also a bit overwhelming because you're looking at how much is there. My therapist has helped me to narrow it down to one thing. There are a lot of techniques I've learned which have been beneficial but it's still difficult.*

Dr X: *Even if it's difficult, what's one thing that helps a little?*

Captain America: *Therapy practices, but it's based on the individual. Some people might not find CBT beneficial.*

Iron Man: *I've noticed you've had times when you've seemed better.*

Captain America: *I don't know if this is Imposter Syndrome, but even if I seem it, I might not feel it. So, it's difficult for me to understand.*

Batman: *What helps me is helping people. Board games. I enjoy people, and being part of this board game community here. I also enjoy playing video games at home. Things like that keep me centred and less prone to dark thoughts.*

Aquaman: *Not to be a broken record but coming here, playing new games. Sometimes it's nice to distract myself.*

Spiderman: *Being more social with friends. Things like watch parties. Being ourselves. Feeling positive about myself.*

Superman: *If I feel I need to centre myself or have a day to myself. To go off by myself. I don't know if I do things consciously. Maybe to mull it over. Digest it, is probably a better term. To digest it and think 'right that's happened' and deal with it and move on. I don't know if I'm squashing it then. But, doing the little things that I do every day to re-centre myself.*

Iron Man: *I like being alone. If I can't get chance to not do anything I'll do that. But hanging out with my daughter. This little girl is my best friend. I'm looking forward to going out when she's older. I want to introduce her to things I like. We sat down and watched a film the other day. She's been a lot of my focus for my mental health. I need to keep my wellbeing for her.*

Dr X: *I think that knowing what's good for you is important because then you can prioritise that.*

Recovery pastimes are more than just hobbies. They are the things you do which calm you, when you need calming. They are the things which excite you, when you need energy. They make you feel good about yourself, when your esteem needs a boost. They are activities which take your difficult emotions and gradually heal them. They can sometimes be used as a distraction, remembering that distraction is good as a short-term strategy not a long-term strategy. They can sometimes be used to energise you. Or connect you. Or focus you. They can stabilise your mood.

Ali talks about bird-watching

'I love watching birds.

At times it feels like a never-ending pub quiz; the birds asking the questions all the time. That flurry of feathers, that distant chirp – what was that? The delicious sense of satisfaction in knowing an answer – or in learning something new!

But much more than this – once I had learnt a few common birds it felt like I'd been gifted a new perspective on the world around me. Suddenly I'd be aware not just that I was walking down a nice green footpath, but that there was a flock of goldfinches nearby or a wren singing from a hidden place. A stop, a wait and I might see something that would have been lost to me.

Through this new perspective, the passing seasons gained a further depth: the reassuring calls of migrating thrushes over my garden in the middle of a cold autumn night; the celebration of the lone robin singing through the winter; the sheer wonder of the millions of feather-light migrants arriving from sub-Saharan Africa in the spring; the quietness of summer.

Common birds have become old friends in whose company I can relax and delight. Whilst the sporadic promise of a rarity – a flash of colour I was not expecting – an unknown song – keeps me always hoping for something new.

Learning, stopping, noticing, appreciating, finding. I simply love it.'

Every few months something new is presented as the panacea to low emotional health. Running, yoga, nature walks, colouring, team sports, painting, dancing, group singing, gardening, horse-riding and various other pursuits have all claimed to be the answer to management and recovery of low emotional health. And I believe in all of them. Not because I'm hopelessly naïve; I know that management and recovery is incredibly hard. But I genuinely do think that these things can be a great part of your Project Recovery. I find that they definitely quicken recovery and make the project more bearable. I call these things recovery pastimes and recommend that everyone finds a pastime to help with their recovery project. Here are some more examples of men talking passionately about the things they love to do.

Joe talks about acting

'My thing is acting. I did a little bit when I was at school but then I just forgot about it. Then when I was in my forties I started looking around for something to do so I could meet new people. I didn't really consider acting till I saw an open audition for a play that I loved, and I decided to go for it. That first time I only went for a small part because I didn't even know if I could act, but I got the part and loved it. After that I caught the bug. Now I do a couple of shows a year if I can. I'm quite reserved in real life and I love being able to pretend to be someone else. My favourite part ever was Bottom, in **Midsummer Night's Dream**. *He's so pushy and over-the-top. One thing I love is the sense of teamwork. I'm not sporty, so I've never really known that sense of working together on something important, but you get that when you work on a play. I've made friends for life through acting.'*

Lee talks about running

'When asked if I could write something about how running helps me manage my own mental health it made me realise that I hadn't given too much thought to it before. On reflection, for me it's more than the well-known release of endorphins that gives that much needed runners-high that is most welcome when we can be feeling low. It's also the satisfaction that I have done something beneficial for myself rather than just do nothing. In my darker times

there have been long periods when even taking a vitamin seemed too much effort but now I can choose to go for a run of over twenty miles, just for fun, just because I can. That gives me a sense of satisfaction and has taken time to get to this point. Viewed over longer terms it has maintained my interest and focus in many areas as I look to improve. Spending time understanding how I can improve my diet, fluids, sleeping patterns, running technique (yes, even at my age LOL), etc., rather than just sit bored which is where negative thoughts can creep in. So I guess some kind of positive distraction in many ways. Not to forget getting plenty of fresh air and the social aspects (on some runs at least LOL), like Parkrun for example. A great way to start the weekend and a habit I would encourage others to start.

My New Year's resolution this year (can't be the only one still doing this can I?) was simply to try to see my glass as half full rather than half empty and new problems merely new opportunities. Think it might be working as rather than get fed up about my recent self-isolation due to a positive Covid test I told myself I probably needed a week off training anyway (one of a number of lessons learned during many YouTube videos – rest can be as important as the training).

So put your trainers on. What are you waiting for? Each run starts with a single step.'

Jordan talks about physical exercise

'One of the biggest challenges for me personally through-out the recent lockdowns were moments where my emotional and mental health felt under pressure. Having times in my life where I wasn't able to engage with the people and activities I love led to that pressure.

One of those important activities in my life has been physical exercise. Being able to play football and go to the gym has given me ways to release difficult emotions.

The physical benefits of feeling fitter, healthier and stronger alongside the chemical reactions whilst my endorphins have been released and the social element of sport all regularly keep my emotional balance in a good space.

Recently, due to a friend's encouragement, I have taken up sea water swimming. During the colder months it is certainly less swimming and more dipping into what feels like freezing cold water and getting out as quickly as possible. The worst moments are when you are first dipping your toe into the water just before you immerse yourself. I have found that after a few minutes of adjusting it's surprising how long we can last. Once the swim or dip is over you feel amazing. Since starting this activity I have noticed my physical and mental health improve, I am sleeping better and I am loving this new hobby. Recently we were joined by a seal swimming only a few feet away from us. What an incredible moment this was for all of us, that never would have taken place if we hadn't tried something new which was slightly outside our comfort zone.

I have come to realise how important physical activity is for me in this season of my life to help rebalance the stress and pressure I face. I have also learnt the importance of making this a part of my regular routine and being as consistent as I can but also forgiving myself if I miss a session because I am busy.

I would recommend to anyone the importance of finding something which helps and supports their emotional and mental health. I am so grateful that one of the ways I do this in my life is through physical exercise.'

I've tried numerous things as part of my own recovery project, and some things have stuck, and others haven't. That's partly for practical reasons, like money, and where I live and what's available, but also for more elusive reasons. Some things

I loved immediately, like gardening, and others I hated but stuck with, like running. In most things I tried I found various features which the activities shared, although various features were stronger in some pursuits than others. I think it's important for people to be able to honestly reflect on what is missing in their lives. If they are going to invest time and energy into a pastime as part of their recovery project, then it is important to try and get a good fit. And the good fit isn't always the thing which you think it will be.

Elements shared by most recovery pursuits.

Purpose

A good recovery pastime has a sense of purpose to it.

Sense of achievement.

A good recovery pastime has achievable aims. Recognising and celebrating these creates a sense of achievement.

Community

A good recovery pastime can eventually bind you to a community. This doesn't always happen straight away, but it can be a good goal to keep in mind.

Connection

A good recovery pastime builds a sense of connection. This could include: connecting to others; connecting to yourself; or connecting with nature.

Flow

A good recovery pastime loses you in its flow. This is when you lose yourself in an activity and everything else fades away.

Commitment

A good recovery pastime builds a sense of commitment. Commitment seems like such a dull thing, but it is incredibly important for recovery.

Self-awareness

A good recovery pastime builds self-awareness. By focusing our attention on a recovery pastime, we can learn things about ourselves that we didn't know. Eventually we might learn to accept our strengths and weaknesses.

Creativity

A good recovery pastime builds creativity. It doesn't need to be a typically 'creative' pastime, but it will help you develop creative ways to tackle the inevitable hurdles.

Consider these elements. Now consider what pastimes fit these parameters.

Without editing yourself, quickly list ten ideas which you could focus on as Recovery Pastimes.
1.
2.
3.
4.
5.
6.

7.
8.
9.
10.

Now look at your list and edit it down to three. Consider what excites you, and interests you. But also consider more practical things.

What is available and what is achievable?
1.
2.
3.

Start with these three pastimes. For now, they can become your recovery pastimes. You can use them to regulate your emotions.

> **KEY POINT:** *Recovery pastimes can help you to regulate your emotions.*

Why do people stall in recovery?

In this next section, we will look at why people can stall in recovery. They have taken the first step, they have started to talk about feelings, they have started to change unhelpful thinking habits, they have recognised that recovery includes 'simple' things which are far from simple, and they've started developing a handful of recovery pastimes. In my experience, there are two connected reasons why recovery can become difficult at this stage.

One reason why recovery can stall at this point is that people find themselves unable to build up a network of support. Help is available, but professional help is hard to access and can take a long time. A person's new interests and recovery pastimes can lead to wider support networks, but this also takes time.

The most important ingredient for a helper is empathy. It is when people show empathy that healing and recovery take place. A support network doesn't need to be huge: a handful of people who are capable of listening with empathy is all that's needed.

Another reason why recovery can stall is that people don't understand the different patterns of recovery. Recovery is never a simple upward line. Recovery is not consistent or predictable. Things get better, and then crash backwards. There are patterns and moods to recovery, and there is some shape to these, once we begin to understand them.

In my experience there are four main phases of recovery. They might overlap or last different lengths of time, but the patterns are usually there. To make recovery easier to understand I have named four common recovery moods after the four seasons.

KEY POINT: *Two common reasons for stalling in recovery are: lack of helpers, and misunderstanding recovery moods.*

Understanding recovery moods

Recovery and management of mental health involves balancing growth and rest. It demands some self-understanding. People need to consider when to push their energies and resources into growth, and when to rest and retreat. Understanding these bodily rhythms is one of the keys to understanding emotional health. Recovery moods are the different stages that people go through in recovery. They don't follow a set pattern, or a set time frame and, although they are named after the seasons, they don't follow the seasons. There is a winter mood, a spring mood, an autumn mood, and a summer mood, but they can come at any time of the year. You can be in a winter recovery mood when the mid-summer sun is streaming through your window. These recovery moods have different purposes.

Winter is for rest and recovery. Spring is for hope and planning. Summer is for growth and creativity. Autumn is for letting go. Every season has a purpose, every season is as important as every other. Recovery can begin in any season of the year, but it often starts in an autumn mood of letting go.

One of the keys to recovery is to listen to your own seasons. They will follow their own rhythm. Some people will rotate round quickly, others much more slowly. When a spring mood comes round, you will feel growth and change and creativity, but just as much is happening when a winter mood takes hold. If the winter mood helps you to find rest and retreat then things are still being achieved, and healing is still taking place.

As you become better at this, the good news is that you spend longer in summer, because you become more efficient at following your own rhythms. This is when recovery can really gain pace. Don't let the set-backs defeat you, they are part of your progress too.

> **KEY POINT:** *Recovery and management of mental health involves balancing growth and rest, and the best way to do this is to understand and follow your recovery moods.*

Letting go (autumn)

Autumn shows us the beauty of letting go. The autumn mood in emotional recovery is a time for talking about feelings and struggles.

What's your favourite thing about autumn?

- Leaves on the trees

- Bonfire night

- Those days when you get warm sun but crisp cold air

- The weather

- Painting the view

- Dark evenings

- Kicking leaves

- New football season.

When I asked people to name their favourite things about autumn, the changing colours of the leaves was by far the most popular answer. We find beauty and comfort in these warm autumnal colours. The trees are getting ready to cast off their leaves. Autumn in nature is about letting go and preparing for rest. The recovery and management of emotional health can begin at any time of the year, but it often starts with an autumnal mood. It often begins by letting go and preparing for rest. This is a time for talking and being listened to.

During the autumn mood we need to find people who will listen to us and open up to them. Open up about feelings, open up about struggles and, if at all possible, open up about things which have made us who we are.

Often during this time of recovery, we begin to grieve for things. Humans grieve for loss and change. Grieving is a process with various stages. Typical stages of grieving are: shock, denial, anger, guilt, bargaining and depression. These stages are moods we work through as we move towards acceptance. Acceptance doesn't mean that we forget what happened, or that it stops hurting, just that we stop fighting against it. As we start to share, we gradually let things go. We can keep their memories, we can keep the things we have learnt, but we need to reach some kind of acceptance. Autumn recovery is about following the rhythms and difficulties of grief before reaching acceptance. There needs to be a lot of talking in the autumn season of recovery. People need to be heard and understood. People can fear different stages of grief, or they can get stuck in one area. It is only by letting go that they can continue to move forward towards a gradual acceptance.

> **KEY POINT:** *The autumn mood is a time for letting go and talking about feelings.*

Rest and recovery (winter)

Winter is a time of comfort. The effort and emotional cost of opening up and talking about things we have held close can be emotionally draining. If we have things to grieve over then this will leave us feeling raw and exposed. In this fragile state we need to embrace comfort, rest and recovery. Just as winter follows autumn, the autumn mood of letting go is followed by the winter mood of rest and comfort. This time of recovery is incredibly important.

What's your favourite thing about winter?

- Christmas
- Open fires
- Knitting
- Pyjamas
- Central heating
- Hot chocolate
- Family time
- Christmas lights.

When I asked people to name their favourite thing about winter, Christmas was the overwhelming favourite. But when I pushed people further, they also talked about open fires, warm lighting, sociable meals with friends, and cosy hot drinks. The Danish have a word for these things – hygge. There are books on hygge, telling us to embrace these comforting behaviours of winter. And I love these ideas and think that hygge is amazing. It is not just when the weather is cold that these things are needed, it is also when we are in a winter recovery mood. Winter recovery moods are the times when we heal our wounds. They are the times when we retreat and hunker down. We need self-care, we need duvet days and the comfort of sadness. Sometimes we need to indulge our inner child and put our own needs first. There are no shortcuts around this. It is so much better to embrace this rather than fight it. If we don't embrace this need for comfort and rest, our bodies and minds often force us into it. Self-care is an essential part of recovery. Winter recovery mood is a frequent visitor. It comes round and round, and continues to heal us. But it isn't forever. One of the reasons why recovery doesn't move forward is that people don't always respond to the healing that takes place. They don't recognise when the time for comfort has led us to a place for moving forward. Rest is for a purpose. It heals. Many people stall in recovery, because they stay in a winter mood. Winter moods are important, but spring should follow winter.

> **KEY POINT:** *The winter mood is a time for comfort and rest.*

Hope and planning (spring)

Spring is a time of new life and creativity. It is a time for hope and recovery and trying new things. It is a time for push and bravery and energy. It is a time for fragile signs of hope. People don't always see the signs of this recovery mood. I would urge people to look for them.

What's your favourite thing about spring?

- Sunshine

- Unexpected warm days

- Long walks

- Weekends away

- Gardening

- New cricket season

- Planning our summer holiday

- Days out.

When spring comes you will sense small moments of hope and expectation bubbling up. You will have days when your mood is clearer and your motivation grows. The key is to take it slowly; summer isn't here yet. You are still fragile, you have a slow season to enjoy. If you take things slowly, then summer will follow.

> **KEY POINT:** *Keep watching for signs of hope and expectation as the spring mood begins.*

Growth and creativity (summer)

Summer can be so beautiful. A summer mood in emotional health is when all your hard work pays off and you feel emotionally connected.

What's your favourite thing about summer?

- Sun

- Holidays

- Family time

- Long evenings with friends

- Camping

- Water fights

- Sailing

- BBQs.

When people go through the letting go of autumn, the comforting self-care of winter, the hope of spring, and then find the growth and creativity of summer, it is an amazing journey.

They find strength in their emotional health. Their emotions become friends. They find things out about themselves and adopt new and healthy rhythms.

People don't stay in a summer mood forever. Our minds and bodies have a way of pacing themselves. We can work things through so successfully that our brains will dig up something else to work through and we go through the journey all over again. If we don't expect this and prepare for it, it can be a real blow to find yourself back in autumn again, preparing to let more things go. This is how our minds and bodies protect us. Things will be worked through piece by piece. This is all progress.

> **KEY POINT:** *Summer moods are times of growth and creativity, but they don't always last forever.*

The cheerleaders and the comforters

Recovery of emotional health is quickened as you build a support network of helpers. It can be hard to find people who listen, but they do exist. It is not just professionals who can listen empathetically. Try talking to a few different people about feelings and see who responds with empathy. These people are gold-dust. Alongside these people, it can be useful to have both cheerleaders and comforters. Some things, and people, inspire you and motivate you and encourage you. These are your cheerleaders. Other things, and people, remind us to rest. They push us towards self-care and comfort. These are your comforters. Both comforters and cheerleaders are helpful at the right times.

If you know where to look, it is relatively easy to find sayings, or real people, who advise us to keep going. Whether they are posters, memes, quotes or people, we can find a hundred different ways for people to tell us to keep going. Some of us even have an internal cheerleader, who keeps urging us on. And sometimes these cheerleaders are the right voice to listen to. Often, they are the best voice to listen to. But they aren't always. Sometimes you have to ignore them.

If you know where to look you can also find some com-forters. These will include sayings, and people who tell us to rest. They will tell us to do the things which make us feel good. And they are right. But they are not always right. Sometimes people listen to their comforters when they need their cheerleaders. And sometimes people listen to their cheerleaders when they need their comforters.

As you think about changing recovery moods, and recognise that recovery involves a balance between growth and rest, rely on your inner voice alongside your cheerleaders and comforters.

> **KEY POINT:** *Sometimes it is right to be encouraged on, and sometimes it is right to seek rest. Listen to your instincts alongside your cheerleaders and comforters.*

PART FOUR

TACKLING THE PROJECT

THE NUTS!

The principles outlined in this book are designed to be useful for dealing with difficult emotions. This involves accepting the fact that we all struggle with difficult emotions from time to time, and all of us have different ways of coping. Some of these ways are healthier than others and some are more effective than others.

The strategies explained in this book are useful to anyone. They include:

- **T**reating difficult emotions as alarm bells
- **H**ealthy life balance
- **E**nding unhealthy habits

- **N**oticing feelings
- **U**sing safe places
- **T**hinking about why you feel that way
- **S**peaking about feelings.

These strategies are always helpful. You could say they are THE NUTS!

> **KEY POINT:** *THE NUTS is an acronym to describe the main principles of this project.*

Treating difficult emotions as alarm bells

In Part Two I use the analogy of driving along a country lane when a warning light comes on. I suggested that a helpful way to understand and deal with difficult emotions is to consider them as warning lights. Difficult emotions are like the warning lights on your car. They don't feel good, but they have a job to do. A similar analogy is that of an alarm.

Consider being alone in a building when an alarm goes off. You aren't entirely sure what the alarm is for.

What would you do?

In the analogy of a warning light on a car, the best decision was to get to a safe place and stop. Similarly, with the alarm, the best decision is to get to a safe place.

The point about alarms is that we need them. They are useful and they have a job to do. This is exactly the same with difficult emotions. They are useful and they have a job to do. Some of us have become so used to fearing, or ignoring, difficult emotions that we actually stop them doing their job. It is a shift of thinking to hesitatingly welcome difficult emotions as reminders to look after ourselves, and to stay safe. When an alarm goes off suddenly and unexpectedly it gives us a momentary panic. This moment of sudden panic doesn't feel great. For a split second we might blame the alarm, especially when it's probably a false alarm. And for a moment we are in fight, flight, freeze mode. Then we realise that it's an alarm and we start using our logical brain to consider if the threat is real. This is exactly how I encourage people to start listening to and using their difficult emotions. Instead of fearing or ignoring the difficult emotion, respond to it, by first getting to a safe place, and then considering if the threat is real, and if there is any way to respond healthily to the threat.

Some people take the batteries out of their alarms. This is the person who has got so used to ignoring or distracting themselves from the difficult emotion that the emotion itself eventually becomes the problem.

> **KEY POINT:** *Try not to fear, or minimise difficult emotions but recognise them as alarms.*

Healthy life balance

I used to think the phrase 'life balance' basically just meant doing less. Then the second lockdown of the Covid pandemic arrived. I'd been lucky enough to receive some furlough during the first lockdown, so I was very well rested already. When I found myself furloughed in the second lockdown my emotional health really slumped. I hated feeling listless and without purpose. I know lots of people had to work through both lockdowns and will have little sympathy for my situation, so I apologise to them, but it really taught me something about life balance. Life balance is so much more than just doing less. I was doing less and less and feeling worse and worse. I was in danger of going into a downward spiral. A lot of wellbeing advice was telling me to rest, but I knew that wasn't what I needed. I needed purpose. Luckily, I noticed the oncoming storm of sustained low mood and I made some deliberate life-changes. I set myself targets, worked on developing new hobbies, made sure I was giving back and generally created purpose for myself.

Life balance isn't just about doing less. We have to regularly consider the balance in our lives between rest and purpose, and this balance changes all the time. It is affected by our health, and energy levels and life circumstances. If we ignore the signals, we can easily tip the scales too far one way, and this is never good for our emotional health.

Consider your balance between rest and purpose.

> *How much of the day is about finding rest, and how much is about purpose?*
>
> *What do the scales usually look like for you?*
>
> *Have you ever known the scales to be balanced?*
>
> *What could you do to bring more balance?*

Life balance in its fullest sense goes further than this. It isn't just about finding the balance between rest and purpose. We also need to consider lots of other elements. Are we taking enough time to self-reflect, or is our focus always on others? Or, is it the other way round? Have we grown so used to thinking about ourselves that we can forget to look outward? Are we so self-critical that it stops us taking risks, or do we have no sense of our own responsibility?

Life balance involves weighing all these elements. It involves taking stock of our situation and our choices and being honest with ourselves.

What areas of your life seem out of balance?

Are there small changes you could make in your life-balance?

How will you apply these changes?

This last question is important, because none of this makes any difference unless you apply these changes. Project Wellbeing involves understanding how to find wellbeing and then applying it to your life.

> **KEY POINT:** *Life balance describes weighing up lots of areas of life and seeing if our priorities need shifting.*

Ending unhealthy habits

One of the breakthroughs in understanding people's emotional health came when I started to think less like an emotional health specialist and more like a gardener. A plant will seek out a healthy life. It will lean towards the sun, it will send down a tap root in its search for water, it will fight pests and diseases to the best of its abilities. When the conditions are not right, or when it becomes overwhelmed, it needs help to become healthy. A healthy plant, like a healthy person, will need certain things in order to flourish.

I'm a keen amateur gardener and I was once given some advice about gardeners which has stayed with me. I was told that there are two types of gardener: those who spend their time and energies directed at the plants, and those who spend their time and energies directed at the soil. Apparently the second group have more success. If you want to succeed as a gardener your best approach is to focus on the soil. When you get that right, healthy plants will naturally follow. This will involve gradually enriching the soil and making it as healthy as possible for the conditions.

I believe in applying the same principles to wellbeing. This involves undoing unhealthy habits of behaviour and thought, and gradually replacing them with healthier habits of behaviour and thinking.

In terms of our physical health, doctors don't heal people, people heal themselves. Doctors may help people identify the right factors for that person's body to seek health, but the patient has to apply them, and the patient's body has to accept them. In mental health the therapists, psychologists and doctors don't heal people, people do. The experts may be able to identify certain factors to help the client to seek health. The client has to apply them. The client has to learn to regulate themselves in certain ways and align themselves to healthy habits.

Noticing and changing habits is a long slow project. Things don't change quickly or easily. One of the most difficult parts of the project is ending unhealthy habits. We've learned them for a reason, and initially they probably brought comfort. They have grown up around us and become ingrained. But there comes a time when the habit itself becomes the problem. In the first two parts of this book I gave some examples of thinking habits which can hold people back from the fullness of emotional health. Things like: pretending to be fine, avoiding talking about feelings, giving up when things become difficult, not seeking help and support, an inability to find a good balance between purpose and rest, becoming defensive when talking about feelings, or always looking for a quick fix.

Can you think of any habits which have become unhealthy for your wellbeing?

When it comes to changing any habit, the first stage is to name it. Consider these examples: pretending to be fine, not talking about feelings, giving up when things become difficult, avoiding help, speeding up through stressful times, looking for a quick fix, turning to drink, drugs, or comfort eating. There will be some of these things which have become habits. Name them, or other unhelpful habits.

The second stage is to become used to noticing them. This sounds easy, but often isn't. That's the thing with habits, we don't always notice them until we deliberately do. Once you have identified an unhealthy habit you need to practise noticing yourself doing it. Name it and call it out.

The next stage is to stop doing it. Some people are able to stop habits in one go. By force of will, they commit to ending the habit in one go. Others need to set gentler targets. With emotional health, these habits have become deeply ingrained and they bring us comfort. Be forgiving with yourself as you start to change these unhealthy habits.

> **KEY POINT:** *Ending unhealthy habits is a long and difficult project, but ignoring them is worse.*

Noticing your feelings

As you think of difficult emotions as alarms, and respond to them, you can get better at noticing them. This is about learning about yourself and recognising your own rhythms. If you struggle with one particular emotion, keep a diary of when you feel that thing, and what things set you off. Allow yourself to notice the emotion.

Notice emotions often but, most importantly, notice them early. The quicker you can notice the presence of difficult emotions the easier they can be to manage.

Consider a difficult emotion which you frequently experience. Write it down.

What does it feel like in your body?

- Stomach: do you get butterflies, or knots in your stomach? Or frequent stomach aches? Do you have a loss of appetite, or food cravings?

- Skin: does your skin get clammy, sweaty, hot or cold?

- Hands: do your fingers clench or curl?

- Toes: do you clench your toes?

- Teeth: do you grind your teeth, or clench your jaw?

- Breathing: does your breathing become faster, heavier or irregular? Or do you struggle for breath?

- Head: do you get headaches?

- Body: do you become fidgety, or need to pace?

- Heart: does your heartrate become faster, heavier, or irregular?

- Chest: do you feel a tightness in your chest?

What does it feel like in your mind?

- Do your difficult feelings affect your sleep?

- Do you notice your difficult emotions before they overwhelm you?

- Do you notice that you become snappy, or grumpy?

- Do you find yourself becoming withdrawn?

- Do you notice that you become difficult to live with?

- Do you sense an increase in negative thoughts?

- Do you have persistent habits connected with your emotional health?

- Do you have mood swings?

- Do you struggle to concentrate?

- Do you feel anxious or panicky?

What are your patterns?

- Are there worse times of the day?

- Are there worse times of the week?

- Are there worse places?

- Are there circumstances which make it worse?

- Are there activities which make it worse?

- Are there people who make it worse?

Look for unusual patterns

The more you start to notice your feelings the more you can begin to spot habits. I never realised that I hummed the theme tune to *Last of The Summer Wine* when I felt anxious. It was my wife who pointed this out to me. Now it's a useful guide to my feelings. Sometimes I start humming before I've even realised that I'm growing anxious. This is like an early warning system for me and helps me to manage my feelings before they grow more difficult.

> **KEY POINT:** *Actively become interested in your emotional world. Look for patterns and habits. Try to spot emotional build-up quickly.*

Using safe places

The project of restoring emotional health includes the use of safe people, safe pastimes and safe places. Safe people are needed as talking about feelings is one of the keys to emotional health. Safe pastimes, or recovery pastimes, are needed because they bring good things such as purpose, self-esteem, calm, structure, creativity and positivity. Safe places are needed because they bring calmness and belonging.

As you begin to notice your feelings, you can also begin to regulate your feelings. Safe places quickly become a cornerstone of this. When you notice your difficult feelings, you get to your safe places as quickly as you can. You allow your safe places to calm you and regulate your emotions.

Safe places bring calm and belonging which help you feel more able to deal with difficult things in your life. As you get used to thinking about your emotions you can then start to think about what causes these difficult feelings.

When I work with people on their emotional health, I ask them to write down three people, three places and three pastimes which help them feel calm. These are your safe places.

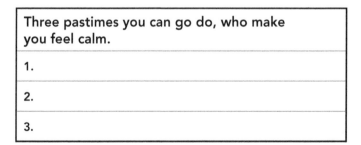

Three people you can talk to, who make you feel calm.
1.
2.
3.

Three places you can go to, who make you feel calm.
1.
2.
3.

Three pastimes you can go do, who make you feel calm.
1.
2.
3.

KEY POINT: *Find people, places and pastimes which help you feel calm and then use them.*

Thinking about why you feel that way

One of the keys to Project Wellbeing is for safe places to have a purpose. Safe places can start out as bunkers, to hide from the difficult feelings of life, but after a while they need to become war rooms, to plan the fight back. As you allow safe places to calm you, there can be a moment when you feel ready to engage with your difficult emotions. At this point you start examining your feelings. What is causing these difficult emotions? This question might seem obvious, but often isn't. Difficult feelings wash over us like a wave, swamping us and making us confused. But every wave is made up of hundreds of droplets. It's the same with difficult emotions. Hundreds of noticed and unnoticed things have built up into that overwhelming feeling. The more things we can name and understand, the more we feel equipped to deal with them. There will be a mixture of things we can do something about, and things we need to let go. Start with the simple things. Are there any causes of our mood which can be dealt with relatively simply? Next, think about things which you would like to let go. Can you let go, or not? Don't fret if you can't; leave those things for another day. Are there any big things which you can chip away at, a piece at a time?

In this way, a safe place becomes a planning area, where emotions are analysed and considered. And sometimes things get dealt with.

Speaking about feelings

There are no magic wands when it comes to dealing with difficult emotions, but speaking about them is as close as you can get to one! Something incredible happens when we get listened to. Firstly, we feel lighter. We actually feel like we've passed on a load. This is always a good thing.

Secondly, we make sense of our own thoughts and feelings as we express them to someone else. Difficult feelings have a habit of tying our thoughts in knots. Talking to someone goes some way to unravelling the knots.

Don't expect people to offer useful advice – they won't. But don't let that put you off. It isn't advice you need, it is empathy. Most people are willing to help but don't always know how. As long as people are empathetic and can listen to you talk, they will help. People who are empathetic will listen without judgement, and they will express some understanding. They may say things like 'that does sound hard'. Empathy is calming and improves our wellbeing.

> **KEY POINT:** *As you reflect on where your difficult feelings are coming from, start to share your feelings with somebody who listens and offers some understanding.*

Project management

Management of emotional health is possible, but it takes work. In this book, the project blueprint is laid out as THE NUTS. Thinking about, and talking about your emotional health is a long-term project. Using THE NUTS model is a long-term project. So you may have to consider project management.

If you wanted to walk a hundred miles, you would need to plan ahead. You would need to plan breaks and rest points on the journey, but you would also have to manage the walk as you went along. You would have to respond to changing conditions and react to circumstances as they come up. You would have times for unscheduled rest breaks, but also times when you push on through and keep going.

My experience of working alongside people as they seek to improve their wellbeing is that they are more successful if they take project management seriously.

We have days when we want to give up when we should probably push through. But we also have days when we dig deep and push through, which can set us back. As you journey with your emotional health, consider recovery seasons, but ultimately the key to the journey is to keep moving in a general direction. Emotional health doesn't come quickly or easily and there will be setbacks, but just keep moving in a general direction and eventually you will be able to look at how far you have come.

Knowing when to seek professional help

Another incredibly important part of project management is knowing when to seek professional help. There are no exact rules when it comes to seeking professional help. This book is about self-care and widening your support network, but you may also need to seek professional help. If so, do so without delay. There is nothing in this book which will contradict with professional advice, and involving experts is an important part of any project.

PART FIVE

PARTICULAR KEYS TO WELLBEING

Men! Check your NUTS!

The principles in this book are designed for all areas of wellbeing. I sincerely believe that learning and applying these principles will always help. Men, you need to be checking your NUTS regularly. These are the cornerstones of this project.

These include:

- **T**reating difficult emotions as alarm bells
- **H**ealthy life balance
- **E**nding unhealthy habits

- **N**oticing feelings
- **U**sing safe places
- **T**hinking about why you feel that way
- **S**peaking about feelings.

These principles remain the same for all areas of emotional health. But certain areas of wellbeing have their own additional quirks which I'd like to explore further.

Sleep

For many people, one of the absolute keys to their wellbeing is improved sleep. Our emotional health struggles and our sleep struggles are connected. Left unchecked they will spiral down a vicious cycle. Sleep struggles affect our emotional wellbeing, and our emotional health affects our sleep. The good news about vicious cycles is that, turned the other way, they can become virtuous cycles. As we improve our emotional health our sleep improves and, crucially, as we focus on our sleep it will help our emotional health. This is why I have started this part of this book with sleep. It's a great place to start improving your overall wellbeing.

Consider the last time you felt fully awake. When was the last time you didn't have a drop of tiredness in your system? Was it today? Yesterday? A week ago? A month ago? There is a significant amount of people who would describe themselves as constantly tired. If that describes you, I empathise. I too have had struggles with sleep.

When did tiredness become so common? When did sleeping become so hard? What have we done to make something which used to be so simple become so complicated? The reality is that sleep was always complicated, but we didn't have to think about it because the conditions for sleep were usually right. For most people now, the conditions for sleep are no longer right, unless we deliberately make them so. In common with all other wellbeing areas in this book, the principle to improving sleep is to improve the conditions around it, and develop healthy habits.

In tackling sleep, we can focus on getting the conditions right, and things will gradually put themselves right. If you focus all your attention on the problem, sleeplessness, we become more aware of the problem, which makes us less likely to sleep well. By focusing on improving sleep conditions we can relax in the knowledge that our sleep patterns will gradually align themselves with new patterns. This approach involves making small changes and allowing time for these changes to make a recognisable impact.

I am going to describe three keys to improved sleep. They are all worth a try; some, or all, of them might improve your sleep and none of them should make your sleep worse.

Sleep difficulties are widespread and chronic and commonplace. Sleep deprivation includes both length of sleep and quality of sleep. Sometimes people get enough hours of sleep, but they still feel tired. Sometimes people can't get to sleep. Sometimes people regularly wake up when they want to be asleep. These sleep problems are significant, but they're not unfixable. Fortunately, although sleep problems are so varied, the solutions are not. The solutions always revolve around creating the right conditions for the sufferer's body to re-learn good sleep patterns.

We all know the signs of tiredness: bags under the eyes, pallid skin, frequent headaches, dry lips, sugar cravings; and that's just when we look at ourselves in the mirror. As someone who has also suffered with sleep deprivation, it took me a while to recognise a crisis even when it was literally staring me in the mirror.

What is sleep?

Imagine an alien race, which didn't sleep, asking what sleep was, what would you tell them? You could describe behaviour changes such as lying down, closing eyes, reducing activity; or you could describe physiological changes such as heart rate slowing, breathing slowing, lowering body temperature and starting to dream. Sleep is when we reversibly disengage with the environment around us, suspend full consciousness, and relax our nervous system. It sounds simple but is actually very complex. Many things happen when we sleep. There are four distinct stages of sleep. In stage 1, 'light sleep', we gradually disengage with the environment. Ideally, we then drift into stage 2, where we generally spend the longest time. During this stage, our brain 'prunes' away unnecessary thoughts and memories as it goes through a daily clean. Stage 3 is deep sleep. During this stage our heart rate slows, our breathing regulates, and our body temperature drops. The last stage is Rapid Eye Movement (REM). During this stage our brains become very active, and produce vivid dreams. In a healthy sleep rhythm, we cycle through these stages four or five times in a night, each cycle lasting between ninety to 120 minutes. So, a good night's sleep will have at least four clear cycles of REM and non-REM sleep.

Five tips to improved sleep

1. Find a soothing night-time routine and stick to it

2. Switch off screens half an hour before bed

3. Avoid eating too late

4. Make sure your bedroom is dark, quiet and cool

5. Write down distracting thoughts before your head hits the pillow

Sleep is important for: memory retention, attention, creativity, insight, problem solving, emotional regulation, emotional balance, growth, healing and building immunity. Each of these areas is developed in different stages of the sleep cycle. REM sleep builds insight and problem solving, by helping to link ideas. It also stores and makes sense of emotions, helping with our emotional regulation. Deep sleep encourages growth and healing and refreshes the immune system. Both REM and deep sleep are needed for memory retention. Sleep is incredibly important, and it's not just length of sleep which matters but quality of sleep as well. It is only in quality sleep that these cycles can fully do their distinct jobs.

Lifestyle Changes

Our culture of busyness, screen addictions, stressful lifestyles and poor emotional health have created a culture of pervasive sleep deprivation. The light of electronic devices, twenty-four hour access to social media, and rising stress and anxiety, exacerbate this problem. To break some of our culture's destructive habits, patterns and behaviours takes effort, understanding and lifestyle changes. Causes of sleeplessness vary from person to person, but busyness, stress, anxiety, poor emotional health, lack of routine, lifestyle choices and technology are often at the heart of things. These societal patterns are not fixed in stone. We have some control over these things. We don't need to be victims of unhealthy cultural behaviours. For most people, tiredness isn't something which has just happened to them. Simple lifestyle changes can reverse sleep deprivation and help us build a fuller and healthier life. Sleep is complicated, and the keys to unlock sleep can vary, but there are one or two things which resonate with most people.

The first is one that most people will recognise. No screens before bed!

We should be switching off screens an hour before sleep. The irony is that lots of people know that and still don't do it. The temptations are too great. When we are lying awake, unable to sleep, the convenience of reading from a device is too strong. This is when some understanding of the science behind sleep can be helpful. When we begin to understand why switching off phones helps us sleep, we are more likely to trust that it can make a difference. Briefly then, five things influence our sleep the most: light, food, temperature, exercise and social interaction. The most important of these is light. Before we sleep, our bodies release melatonin, which is then broken down by morning light. When we use smartphones and tablets before sleep, it completely disrupts this process. This is the part that some people know, and some will use a night-light feature. These night-light features will usually help a bit, but not enough. What people don't know is that even a switched-off connected device can still disrupt sleep. Think back to those five factors which most influence sleep. One of them is social interaction. Think about how awake you feel at a party, or on a good night out with friends. Social interaction keeps us awake, and our brains associate our connected devices with social interaction. Researchers found that the use of screens before bed doubled the chances of a disrupted sleep. But, crucially, they found that sleep disruption was only fractionally less when people had phones with them in the room, even if they were switched off.[1]

Our brains associate screens with social interaction, and when screens are nearby we become reluctant to switch down. If you have a connected device in your room, it is like knowing that there's a great party happening in your house which you are trying to sleep through. Even if you do fall asleep, your quality of sleep will be affected as your brain remains alert. Sleeping well is not just about the hours you get, but how effective this sleep is.

---

1 (http://www.telegraph.co.uk/science/2016/10/31/smartphones-and-tablets-in-bedrooms-disrupt-sleep-even-when-swit/)

KEY ONE: switch off phones before bed.

A second key is quiet before sleep. Our busy lifestyles and constant access to screens and social interaction keep our brains alert for extended periods of time. Our brains have evolved to want periods of alert and periods of calm. Many things happen in the calm periods, and one of these things is that our brains reflect and review, as well as organise things to be aware of. In other words, our brains will sort things out and organise. We often forget to deliberately include these periods of calm in our schedules, so our poor brains will grab the first opportunity they can – often the minute our head hits the pillow. The first time our brains receive the calmness they crave is just as we expect them to quieten down. Our brains then refuse to calm down as they've got important work to do. I have lost count of the amount of people who complain that worries keep them awake. It is literally in the hundreds. And yet there is such an easy fix which works for most people. If you reflect on the day quietly before your head hits the pillow you will regain some control over your wayward thoughts.

KEY TWO: a quiet reflective time before bed.

Sleep quality is affected by our circadian rhythms. Five things influence our circadian rhythms: light, food, temperature, exercise and social interaction. Our sleep quality is highest when these five factors – light, food, temperature, exercise and social interaction – work together to promote good sleep. When all these things work together to strengthen our circadian rhythms, we will sleep well, but when some things work against these factors we disrupt our natural rhythms.

The absolute best way to prepare the body for sleep is to have a routine. Consider the five factors which affect the circadian rhythms – light, food, temperature, exercise and social interaction. Find a way to gradually switch each one down in a regular night-time routine, and stick with it. One thing that I do is gradually lower the volume of TV or music, starting over an hour before bed.

KEY THREE: develop a routine and stick to it.

These three quick fixes are good examples of how to approach these problems. The lifestyle changes needed to tackle sleeplessness are both simple and complicated. They look simple, because they are easy to explain. But they are also complicated because they involve lifestyle changes and consistency. These things only start to work when they become ingrained habits.

The perfect sleep environment

- Build a routine. Get used to going to bed at roughly the same time each night.

- No screens before bed. No electronic devices for one hour before bed.

- Do a series of calming activities before bed. Build these activities into your routine.

- Do you need ear plugs or eye-masks?

- Make your bed a sacred sleep space. Don't do work, screen-time or other non-calming activities on your bed.

- Consider temperature. Cold face, warm toes is best.

- Drinking – no caffeinated drinks at night. Drink things which promote sleep such as non-caffeinated milky drinks, chamomile tea and cherry juice.

- Eating – eat your evening meal at least four hours before bed. Eating raises the body's core temperature which disrupts sleep. Eat protein rich foods, as these boost melatonin.

- Being well exercised – exercise helps with stage 3 sleep

- Have ONE pillow which is right for you.
  - *side sleepers – full and fluffy, medium-high thickness*
  - *stomach sleepers – airy, thin, soft and mouldable*
  - *back sleepers – medium firm, possibly memory foam*
  - *allergy sufferers – synthetic fillings such as polyester or memory foam*

KEY POINT: *Sleep is important for wellbeing. Three keys to improved sleep can be: phone break before bed, rest in the day, routine.*

Rest

It might seem odd to have a chapter on rest, right after a chapter on sleep. Some people think that sleep IS rest. It's not. Good rest during the day will improve sleep. When I talk about good rest, I'm not talking about accidently falling asleep, I'm not even talking about naps at all, but times when the body and mind get the chance to properly switch off. For many people, a key to improving their wellbeing is to focus on developing deliberate and effective rest.

The interesting thing about rest is that it's always a condition of health. Always. What do doctors always tell us to do? What do our bodies always crave when they're ill? Rest! How can we possibly think that mental health is any different? There might be lots of specific things we need, but these will always include rest.

I've been thinking a lot about rest recently. How can I rest better? I don't think it's just about having more rest, but having more effective rest.

For the past year I've been doing a painting a day, and I have been describing these daily moments of focused calm as islands. Sometimes life can seem like an exhausting sea that we constantly swim through without pausing to enjoy the moment. My daily paintings are the times in every day when I pause and enjoy the moment. What has been amazing about my daily paintings is that they bring both purpose and rest in the same activity. I don't paint to achieve anything, I paint for my wellbeing, but it's a nice bonus when I create something I'm proud of. I love creativity, and creative rest is one of the joys of life for me. I believe that creative rest is for everyone, regardless of any false ideas about talent. But creative rest is only one form of rest. There are many shapes of rest.

- **Physical Rest.** Sometimes we need to rest our bodies. Developing good sleeping habits helps with this. Sometimes we need to use our bodies to rest our minds. Physical rest helps us re-charge.

- **Creative Rest.** Creative rest helps us find the sweet spot between purpose and rest. No talent is required but it can be useful to find your inner child and re-kindle your sense of wonder and delight. Creative rest helps us re-awaken.

- **Nature Rest.** Letting nature help us to feel rested. Being out in nature helps us to feel part of the world.

- **Spiritual Rest.** Spiritual rest helps us see beyond our own minds and bodies and feel a sense of the other. Anything which helps us feel that there is more to life than meets the eye. Spiritual rest helps us find purpose.

- **Emotional Rest.** Taking time to listen to your own emotions. Listening truthfully to our own feelings and allowing them to do their purpose. Some people might find this easier with a close confidant. Others can use self-reflective activities. Emotional rest helps us understand ourselves.

- **Sensory Rest.** Intentionally giving our senses a break from the noise, lights and information overload we get, particularly from screens. This can involve some lifestyle changes for some people, including screen breaks and no-screen days. Sensory rest helps us to remember who we are.

- **Social Rest.** Enjoying your own company. Enjoying solitude. For some this comes easily, for others it takes practice. But social rest can take another form too. Some of us find rest in other people's company. Particularly with close supportive friends. Social rest helps us re-connect.

- **Mental Rest.** Enjoying the moment. Not planning, remembering or over-thinking. This can take practise. Use mindfulness. Use physical activity. Use anything which helps you lose yourself in the moment. In mental rest we switch off our distracting thoughts. Mental rest helps us to just be.

This isn't a definitive list, and I've seen other lists, some shorter and some longer, but it's a reasonable summary of styles of rest. There's no order to it; it's just a reminder that effective rest can take practice. But, through my year of painting, I have learned to do thirty minutes of focused, intentional rest every day. That's every day. And it has had more impact on my wellbeing than any other single thing. I have learned to prioritise rest, and the reason I do it is to feel more alive. In the last two years I have felt more alive, had more energy, slept better and generally been happier than at any other time in my life. Rest has been key to this.

When I can't find rest

There are times when I can't rest effectively. I'm just too wired to rest well. I've had to learn to see these times as their own particular alarm bells.

I can tell when my work/life balance is good because it's then that rest comes easily to me. At times of high stress, and ridiculous busyness, I run on adrenalin. During these times I know I should rest, but I can't quite settle into it, and it brings no satisfaction.

When our daily rhythms of rest are unbalanced, we find it harder to access effective rest. Consider the first few days of a holiday; it takes us half the first week to remember how to rest. This is why busy people often find rest boring, rather than restful. To me that's a reminder to develop more effective rest by building it into our daily rhythms. This effective rest will then always increase our wellbeing.

> **KEY POINT:** *Rest is important for wellbeing. Daily, focused, intentional rest can hugely improve our wellbeing.*

Stress

One of the things which can make both sleep and rest harder to find is stress. Tackling stress is an effective key to improving overall wellbeing.

'I'm not at all stressed,' said no man ever. It sometimes feels like every adult male I know is carrying too much stress. But, like every other wellbeing area in this book, it's not completely outside of your control. It is something which can be understood and approached like a long-term project.

Stress is your body's way of telling you that you are reaching maximum capacity to cope with things. Like other wellbeing issues, it's like a warning light on your car, telling you to pull over. When you perceive a threat, your nervous system responds by releasing a flood of stress hormones which rouse the body for emergency action. These chemicals include adrenalin and cortisol. These chemicals make your heart beat faster, your muscles tighten, your blood pressure rise, your breath quicken and your senses become sharper.

Some of these physical changes increase your strength and stamina, speed your reaction time and enhance your focus – preparing you to either fight or flee from the danger at hand. Some are ways in which your body tries to ignore irrelevant details and focus on the main danger, and some are just bad habits.

Stress isn't always bad. In small doses, it can help you perform under pressure and motivate you to do your best. Feeling nervous before an interview or presentation can focus your thoughts and help you perform well. A healthy relationship with stress involves a balance of *stress* and *relaxation* in your life. After a stressful thing, you need something to relax you and get rid of the stress chemicals.

Consider how you find rest. After the last chapter, you should already be considering ways to rest more effectively. During stressful times you will need to use these techniques more. Your rhythms of life may need to change with even more deliberate rest periods. In this way you will be getting the most out of both rest and stress.

Sometimes to achieve this balance we need to RECOG-NISE and MANAGE stress. There are particular times of life when stress is inevitable. Times of life with big life changes, for example, such as moving house, leaving school, sitting exams, or job changes. Or times when big decisions need to be made, such as considering career or relationship changes. For a few months you may be constantly running in emergency mode, and there is a chance that your mind and body will pay the price unless you find ways to recognise and manage the stress during this period.

How much stress is 'too much' differs from person to person. We're all different. But if you are experiencing more than one or two of the following factors you may be experiencing 'too much' stress:

- Moodiness

- Feeling overwhelmed

- Sense of loneliness and isolation

- Depression or general unhappiness

- Inability to concentrate

- Seeing only the negative

- Anxious or racing thoughts

- Diarrhoea or constipation

- Nausea and dizziness

- Chest pain and rapid heartbeat.

If you feel you're experiencing too much stress, then you probably are.

Managing Stress

Things that can help lower your stress include:

- **Support network** – A strong network of supportive friends and family members can help. Are you talking about how you're feeling to one or two supportive people?

- **Sense of control** – It may be easier to take stress in your stride if you feel in control of things. As well as talking about your feelings, perhaps someone could help you organise the things which are causing you stress.

- **Emotions** – You're more vulnerable to stress if you don't know how to calm and soothe yourself when you're feeling sad, angry, or overwhelmed. In normal life it is good to find things which calm you down and do them daily. During particularly stressful times you may need to do them more regularly and for longer.

- **Avoid** unnecessary stress. Not all stress can be avoided, but by learning how to say no, and steering clear of people or situations that stress you out, you can eliminate many daily stressors.

- **Alter** the situation. If you can't avoid a stressful situation, try to alter it. Be more assertive and deal with problems head on. Let others know about your concerns.

- **Adapt** – When you can't change the stressor, try changing yourself. Focus on the positive things in your life.

- **Accept** the things you can't change. There will always be stressors in life that you can't do anything about. Particularly stressful times are difficult, but they shouldn't last forever.

- **Pay attention to other things** – If you need to control stress quickly in a given situation you could try a simple technique of using your senses. What can you see and hear around you? Look at a favourite photo or smell something comforting, listen to a favourite piece of music or focus on the taste of something you enjoy.

> **KEY POINT:** *Rest is important for wellbeing. Daily, focused, intentional rest can hugely improve our wellbeing.*

Anger

Stress, sleeplessness and lack of rest can make us prone to anger and irritation. These things aren't surprises, and yet sometimes we refuse to acknowledge them. One of my difficulties is when most of men's complicated emotions get labelled and dismissed as anger. I don't think this reductive attitude helps anyone. But out-of-control anger can be a problem for some men, as it can be for anyone.

Anger isn't wrong. Anger is one of our most primitive defence mechanisms. It protects us from being dominated or manipulated by others. It gives us the added strength, courage and motivation needed to combat unfairness done to us or to those we love. Anger is often stronger in people who want things to be fair but who see things that aren't. The urge to seek justice and fairness is a great one, but in many of us our anger gets in the way of finding solutions to things. It overwhelms us and clouds our judgement.

If people act in the heat of the moment their emotions can take control of their actions and they are *less* likely to achieve what they want. Losing your temper can make you feel out of control and powerless just when you most want to feel in control and powerful. Anger becomes a problem when it harms the person expressing it or the people around them. This can depend on whether they express their anger and how they express it.

Anger is an energy. It is a boost to our adrenaline levels, making us feel stronger and more in control. When we can control the anger, this is a good thing. It is a useful survival strategy. Anger is part of our fight or flight response system.

CASE STUDY: **TOM**

Tom is thirteen and angry. I met him on a residential activity weekend and liked him straight away. He was funny and personable but clearly had underlying anger issues. In terms of emotional health I felt that he probably did experience a range of emotions but was worried anger might dominate his life and possibly make it difficult for him to balance his emotions. As he opened up to me I discovered that he was on his third school in that academic year and that he had first been expelled from school at nine. This made me wonder how he expressed his anger and I felt that it was unlikely that he expressed it appropriately. Within a few hours we found out. The first flash-point came when one of the leaders tried to take an E-cigarette off him as he was appearing to share it with other boys. Without listening to any discussion he ran to his room, grabbed a bag and ran away. Fortunately we were staying in the middle of nowhere so despite our extensive efforts to find him he eventually made his own way back. Sometime later he broke a chair when a similar thing happened. And then later the next day he ran away again. On this occasion I managed to walk some distance behind him until he gave up trying to outpace me and decided to talk instead. He told me about various issues, including an absent father, which had caused a build-up of resentment in his life. But the thing he talked about most was the initial incident at the primary school which saw him kicked out. After that, in his mind, he was forever labelled as a troublemaker. He was adamant that he had not done the thing that he was initially accused of. For so many teenagers their anger stems from a feeling of injustice.

Tom's life was being dominated by his anger. After listening to him for some time I had a real sense that the root cause of the anger was an incident from a few years ago which had never been properly explored. I encouraged Tom by telling him how much good he had brought to that weekend with his humour and personality. I then encouraged him to explore what happened in primary school by talking to his family about it. I wasn't in a position to know whether his injustice was real or perceived but I felt that if he could talk it through calmly with his family he might feel better when some of his real grievances were aired. I told him how important it was to deal with this one small thing in his life because he had so much else to offer.

When you don't express your anger, or express it at inappropriate times, or in unsafe ways, it can damage your health, your relationships and your wellbeing. This is especially so if something has made you angry in the past and you didn't express your anger at the time – because you felt you couldn't or didn't want to – then that anger can get 'bottled up' or 'suppressed'. This can have negative consequences in the long term – you may find that when something happens to annoy or upset you in the future, you feel extremely angry and respond more aggressively than is appropriate to the new situation.

When people spend their whole time fighting their anger, rather than managing their anger, they find that they can't get rid of it. When people try to suppress their anger, it pops out in destructive ways.

Anger Management

Anger management involves learning ways to control your anger and direct it constructively. It often involves putting some time and space between the inflammatory situation and dealing with it. By walking away, counting to ten, or using some other technique, you are waiting to act until the anger is more controllable. In this way, the anger is more likely to achieve the result you want.

- **Recognise it.** Anger management involves recognising early signs of anger and taking steps to deal with the situation constructively. Something is causing the build-up of anger, and as we start to recognise our feelings earlier we can see if we can do anything positive to make changes. Anger doesn't have to reach maximum. As we learn to notice the early signs of anger we can take action while anger is in the early stages.

- **Talking.** Talking, and being listened to empathetically, can move the rage and stress from the fight and flight control centre into the higher thinking brain, where we can rationalise it.

- **Walk away.** When our rage reaches a certain level we need to accept that the only thing to do is walk away or count to ten until our feelings simmer down a bit.

- **Become assertive.** Assertive behaviour is based on the belief that your wants and needs are important, but not more so than the wants and needs of others. It is an alternative to aggressive behaviour, which stems from the belief that your wants and needs are more important than others, and to unassertive behaviour, which stems from the belief that your wants and needs are less important than those of other people.

- **Reflect.** Anger management involves reflecting on what the specific triggers are which stimulate passionate emotions. What is at the root cause of our anger, and also what specific things trigger it?

Anger management is a skill to be practised repeatedly, becoming easier each time. We make mistakes, and lose control but we keep practising anger management because eventually we learn to control the anger, rather than letting the anger control us. Some people fear that if they manage their anger the world will walk over them, but the opposite is the case. It is only when we learn to manage anger that we can get the results which we want.

The point of managing anger is to place yourself in control of the anger, rather than allowing the anger to control you. Most ways of managing anger have in common one thing, take time out. The reason for this is to cool off. This is so that you can look inward first and react to the actual cause of the anger and not the feelings inside. When you have calmed down you will be better equipped to deal with whatever caused your feelings in the first place. It can be hard work to break your anger habits but ultimately it will make you more in control of fixing the things which made you angry in the first place.

> **KEY POINT:** *Anger isn't wrong but being out of control is harmful. Learning ways to manage anger effectively is a key to wellbeing.*

Depression

Problems with our wellbeing can cause us to feel depressed. Every day, several times a day, I help people who struggle with difficult emotions. As you'd expect, a large part of that is helping people who struggle with depression. Some mental health conditions are more manageable than others, and depression undoubtedly falls into the difficult category. When I workshop emotional health, I ask people to name emotions, and then put them in order from most pleasurable to most difficult. Depression and Grief are frequently placed at the far end of difficulty.

The principles at work in this book can help people in the management of depression, and there's nothing that I wouldn't stand by as being useful in understanding and learning to manage depression.

These include: having some sense of control over your emotions, seeing it as a long-term project to develop healthier habits and practices, having realistic targets in mind, talking, recovery pastimes, rest, self-care. If there is one big difference, I'd hesitatingly suggest that it might be in accepting that the project may be a longer and more involved one. But the principle of seeing the management of wellbeing as a long-term project remains.

Symptoms of depression vary from person to person and can affect people differently according to their age and gender, but they are often characterised by severe feelings of hopelessness.

Depression can affect people differently, but symptoms can include:

- Feelings of hopelessness
- Low self-esteem

- Lack of focus
- Low energy levels
- Sleeping difficulties
- Lack of appetite
- Comfort eating
- Self-harm
- Reliance on unhealthy habits
- Lack of self-care
- Suicidal thoughts.

Those who are experiencing a combination of these symptoms for two or more weeks should seek medical assistance. GPs are a good first port of call.

Depression is common. It is also feared and misunderstood. I know mental health groups who hesitate to use the word depression and talk instead of 'sustained low mood'. I understand this, and can see a lot of benefit in this. I let the client choose their own terms, but I can see why the word depression can make people feel less likely to think they have any control over their own wellbeing. We've come to see depression solely as a medical issue, but like all mental health issues it's never ALL one thing. There are still things that the individual can do. After seeking medical help, the individual should ideally still feel some sense of autonomy on how to approach their own recovery. Talking things through with an empathetic listener is still the greatest healer. Just as in other mental health states the practice of talking through difficult feelings still helps to move the feelings of hopelessness from the fight or flight response centre in the amygdala, to the clever thinking brain. In addition, developing healthy practices and recovery pastimes, alongside rest, purpose and self-care, will all help.

Depression's Catch-22

If all this is true, then the obvious question remains of why depression can be more persistent. Why is it that tackling depression often becomes a longer-term and more complicated project to undertake? What if you practise all these good things and it barely touches the sides of the depression? To understand this involves two further discussions – recognising depression as a grief stage and recognising depression's catch-22.

We talked about the catch-22 of emotional health in Part 3. Low emotional health drains your motivation, when motivation is the very thing you need to improve emotional health. This circle is present in all examples of emotional ill-health, but it is the defining feature of depression. People with depression can't just decide to stop feeling down. Depression can trap people in a very real and all-consuming catch-22. Depression drains people's motivation, but motivation is the very thing they need to tackle depression. In depressed individuals, there is a fundamental impairment in areas of the brain which support motivation, energy and hope. This makes it more difficult to recover without help. The things a person needs to do to recover are the very things which the illness makes it difficult to do. The person's brain works against their recovery.

An understanding of this catch-22 can help. It can highlight the journey ahead and show what steps can be undertaken, even if those steps seem impossible. It can also help the individual to be kind to themselves and avoid putting additional pressure on their own shoulders. It can also help people to see that small steps will help, even if these things seem annoyingly simple in themselves. Some relatively simple ideas can help with depression, but that doesn't make them simple to do. They still take effort and motivation which are in short supply. These 'simple' things unsurprisingly include: talking, healthy habits, recovery pastimes, rest, purpose and self-care.

The illness makes these things difficult, but not impossible. Sometimes you need to break each one of these things into smaller steps before you can even get a foothold into starting them.

Depression as a Grief State

Another complication with depression is that it is ALSO a natural part of our grieving process. It has been well documented that a mother who has lost a child will fulfil all the checklist factors of depression. But we would rightly call that grief. There is no picking apart the boundaries between depression as an illness and depression as part of the natural grieving process. And yet, it's incredibly important that we do recognise a boundary.

Grief is not just a response to death. We grieve all loss and change in our lives by going through various emotional states. Depression is one of these ways in which we gradually learn to accept loss and change. It is incredibly common to get stuck on this stage. Sometimes people confuse acceptance with forgetting and subconsciously refuse it. Or they are just not ready to move on. In these circumstances, depression can feel destructive and hopeless, but is part of our natural healing process. When we hold the depression inside it can block us, but if we talk openly about these feelings than the brain can move onwards through the grieving process.

Grief is natural and healthy and purposeful. Sometimes depression is an illness but sometimes it is part of the grieving process. Depression as part of the grieving process is still painful, and horrific, but it has a job to do.

> **KEY POINT:** *Remember that Depression is OFTEN a natural part of the grieving process.*

Anxiety

Anxiety is my constant companion. But, because I regularly manage my emotional health, I am rarely held back by it. It feels strange to say it, but it has virtually no negative effects on my life these days.

Anxiety is a feeling of unease. Everyone has feelings of anxiety at some point in their life – when attending an interview or getting married, for example. During times like these, feeling anxious is perfectly normal.

Anxiety can feel like:

- Restlessness

- Worry which won't go away

- A feeling of emptiness in your stomach

- Heart palpitations

- Shortness of breath

- Racing thoughts

- Overthinking

- Negative thoughts

- Dizziness

- Light-headedness

- Sweating

- Nausea

- Frequent trips to the bathroom

- Feelings of detachment

- Difficulty concentrating.

The feelings in the tummy, and the heart palpitations, are because your brain is redistributing its resources by moving more blood to your brain. The restlessness, sleeplessness and worry are because your brain won't let you ignore it.

Five unusual ways to feel less anxious

- Stand on one leg (there is actual scientific evidence that this can lower anxiety!)

- Gently rub your lips (this too… I'm not kidding!)

- Watch a film that makes you sad

- Take a walk with a great view

- Sing loudly to a favourite song

Anxiety is a response to threat. Your amygdala has noticed a threat to your world and is warning you. It could be a physical threat, like fear of heights, or an emotional threat like social anxiety, the fear of being made fun of. Very often, low level feelings of anxiety are simply a normal reaction to stress. This can be a good thing. Anxiety can help motivate you to accomplish things in your life that are important to you, or it can warn you to focus hard on something, or it can stop you forgetting certain details.

When is anxiety a problem?

Some low-level anxiety is normal and controllable. But, for many people, anxiety can become problematic and seemingly uncontrollable. People learn to cope with anxiety by avoiding things, people or situations. Anxiety becomes a problem when it negatively impacts everyday life.

Anxiety can become a problem if:

- It stops you enjoying everyday life
- It causes you to avoid certain situations
- It's clearly disproportionate to the severity of the threat
- There is no obvious threat.

In common with other wellbeing issues in this book, it can be helpful to think of anxiety as an alarm bell ringing in your mind, shouting at you over and over not to ignore it. It's entirely possible that nothing alarming is actually happening, but your brain has decided that there is. This is when anxiety can become a problem. Most people have a baseline level of anxiety, where they naturally gravitate to. People who are rarely anxious will have a low baseline or background level of anxiety. They might rarely feel worried or anxious. But many people get so used to background worry that their baseline level of anxiety is already high, even when there is no perceivable threat. Their brains become finely tuned to threats in everyday life and that nagging feeling of worry rarely, if ever, goes away. In the alarm analogy, picture an alarm which has become too sensitive and goes off all too often. I have a smoke alarm like this which goes off whenever I cook bacon. Sadly, the temptation in the moment is just to smash up the alarm rather than find ways to make it less sensitive.

CASE STUDY: **ALEX**

Alex was a happy child, but had a difficult transition to Secondary School. His friends went to another school and they found themselves in a class where they didn't know anyone. His first attempts at making friends didn't go very well. He found himself in a group of bullies, who were mean to him. School became a daily threat to his emotional and physical safety. He became withdrawn and stopped trying to make friends. This made things worse as he found himself without any safe places within the school. He started skipping school, but this became unsustainable, so he started faking illness. This only lasted so long until he had to go back to school. Every time he tried avoidance it seemed to make things worse. He tried to turn up to school daily, but kept his head down and avoided eye-contact. This made him very self-conscious. He started to feel the physical symptoms of anxiety, including a racing heart and increased sweating. He was still being bullied so he joined an after-school art class to avoid the bullies on the walk home. Fortunately, this is where things started to change. Amongst a small group in the art class he began to make some friends. In addition, the safe space in the school helped to calm him down and he was allowed to visit the class at other times in the school day. He also developed a talent for art and poured some of his negative thoughts into this creative activity. He was asked to paint a mural on a school wall. Although it was a long way out of his comfort zone he embraced the opportunity. This led to further opportunities and his anxiety gradually became manageable. He still uses art as a way to manage his anxiety as an adult.

Many problems with anxiety are not based on our fears, but on our struggles with anxiety itself. If you think of anxiety as a match, when it has done its work it blows itself out. But when you get stuck in an anxiety loop it doesn't go out. It then flares up (e.g. panic attacks) or continues to smoulder (e.g. free-floating anxiety or anxiety disorders). People can then feel hounded by emotions they can't get rid of. Recognising these issues can give you a foothold into managing them. If your baseline anxiety is high, it is when there are no obvious threats that you can be working on calming techniques. People often only work on calming techniques in the throes of high anxiety, but it is just as important to work on habits of calm in everyday life.

- Ways to manage anxiety

- Understand. Recognise and understand it. WHEN you calm down, analyse it and find the cause of the alarm.

- Drop the baseline. Learn ways to calm down which work for you. Use these regularly and habitually, regardless of where your anxiety levels are.

- Gradually learn to intervene early.

- Know your safe spaces and use them.

- Use a worry diary nightly.

- Speak to people about your feelings.

- Face your fears. When you can, it is important to do the things which cause you worry to break the cycle of avoidance.

> **KEY POINT:** *It can be helpful to think of anxiety as an alarm which, for some people, has become over-sensitive. Doing calming things even when the alarm isn't ringing can reduce your background anxiety.*

Pandemic grief

The world changed in 2020. The repercussions of this pandemic will be with us for many years. As I write this, no one knows how this will end, or how long it will last. The pandemic has had a huge impact on our wellbeing. It was always hard to find wellbeing, but it's even harder in these times.

One day we will grieve these times. Many of us already do. As described elsewhere in this book, grief is a series of emotional states we go through as we adjust to a new reality. This is the reality of life for many people in these times. These times feel chaotic, and they are made even more chaotic as we are in the depths of grief. The world has changed and humans adjust to change slowly, by grinding through various grief stages, often in a chaotic order, and often with more than one grief stage assaulting us at the same time.

Our brains have a pattern for coping with change. The seven commonly recognised stages of grief are:

- Shock

- Denial

- Guilt

- Anger

- Bargaining

- Depression

- Acceptance.

If humans were robots, we would all be programmed to work calmly through each stage in a set order for a set amount of time. We would then emerge fully adjusted into the acceptance stage; but we're not robots. Nowhere near. We adjust to change like we grieve – messily, noisily, chaotically and painfully. This is a period of adjustment, and response to change. Most of us are probably bouncing around various mental states. Our brains don't really understand what is happening, or why, or how to adjust to these changes. In such an unsettled state we are whizzing around the stages of grieving at an unprecedented rate. Some days our brains will be channelling guilt, another day anger. Some days we will find acceptance. With any kind of grief, it is important to allow your brain to feel what it feels.

> **KEY POINT:** *We will grieve the changes brought about by Covid for many years. Grief can be messy and unpredictable.*

Conclusion

There are many voices in this book: paragraphs where people talk about what helps them; transcripts of open conversations with some great people who open up about their struggles; lists of answers to questionnaires. I'm really grateful to all these men, and I hope by including lots of voices I've created a feeling of camaraderie. I want this book to be a safe space where it's ok to not be ok.

I like the expression 'it's ok to not be ok' and I use it a lot. It creates a safe space where people can begin to be open about their emotional struggles. And traditionally men have generally been less open about their emotions than women. Feeling safe to open up about emotional struggles is a great starting point. And it's still a starting point which needs to be made more accessible. Particularly for people who don't know how to open up about their feelings, many of whom are male. It's a great starting point, but it is still just a starting point. My experience of helping people find wellbeing is that, after opening up about struggles, they want to believe in some kind of progress. Management and recovery of emotional health is possible. It's not easy, and improvement is never linear; it comes in bursts of improvement and then times of stasis or regression. Over time things can improve, and this book has explained one model and one process which has had a lot of success. I'm not pretending it's the only model or the only process, but it is a good place to start. The model I've outlined in this book asks people to check THE NUTS:

Treating difficult emotions as alarm bells

Healthy life balance

Ending unhealthy habits

Noticing feelings

Using safe places

Thinking about why you feel that way

Speaking about feelings.

Using this model regularly and purposefully should bring some sense of improvement in emotional health and wellbeing.

> **KEY POINT:** *Check THE NUTS.*

Acknowledgements

n some way all the men I've met have contributed to this book. I particularly want to thank men who have been good role models. We all need good role models in our lives, and I've been particularly lucky with mine. I have known many men who have shown me great examples of how to be a good man.

I particularly want to thank all those men who took a risk and agreed to talk openly about their mental health. I recognise what a brave and beautiful thing that is to do. I want to thank the brilliant men who gathered at Idle Games in Paignton one Sunday evening, lured by free pizza. Mark, Josh, Gary, Paul, Connor, James and Dan, thank you for being open, interesting and brave.

I also want to thank all the men who talked openly and passionately about their hobbies and recovery pastimes. Lee Alsopp, Ali King and Jordan Williams. It was great to include your words about things you are passionate about.

Then there were all the men who took time to fill in a questionnaire with all manner of questions and topics as I reached the net far and wide to gather lots of different opinions from people from many different backgrounds. Tim Funnell, Dave Woods, Ali King, Richard Eley, Dr. Ben King and others. Men who demonstrate that you can choose many different ways to be a great person and a great man.

Thanks, all.